Alzheimer's

The Latest Assessment And Treatment Strategies

George T. Grossberg, MD

The Samuel W. Fordyce Professor
Director of the Division of Geriatric Psychiatry,
Saint Louis University School of Medicine
St. Louis, MO

Sanjeev M. Kamat, MD

Staff Psychiatrist,
Saint Alexius Hospital and Forest Park Hospital
St. Louis, MO

JONES AND BARTLETT PUBLISHERS
Sudbury, Massachusetts
BOSTON   TORONTO   LONDON   SINGAPORE

World Headquarters

Jones and Bartlett Publishers
40 Tall Pine Drive
Sudbury, MA 01776
978-443-5000
info@jbpub.com
www.jbpub.com

Jones and Bartlett Publishers
Canada
6339 Ormindale Way
Mississauga, Ontario L5V 1J2
Canada

Jones and Bartlett Publishers
International
Barb House, Barb Mews
London W6 7PA
United Kingdom

Jones and Bartlett's books and products are available through most bookstores and online booksellers. To contact Jones and Bartlett Publishers directly, call 800-832-0034, fax 978-443-8000, or visit our website, www.jbpub.com.

Substantial discounts on bulk quantities of Jones and Bartlett's publications are available to corporations, professional associations, and other qualified organizations. For details and specific discount information, contact the special sales department at Jones and Bartlett via the above contact information or send an email to specialsales@jbpub.com.

The authors, editor, and publisher have made every effort to provide accurate information. However, they are not responsible for errors, omissions, or for any outcomes related to the use of the contents of this book and take no responsibility for the use of the products and procedures described. Treatments and side effects described in this book may not be applicable to all people; likewise, some people may require a dose or experience a side effect that is not described herein. Drugs and medical devices are discussed that may have limited availability controlled by the Food and Drug Administration (FDA) for use only in a research study or clinical trial. Research, clinical practice, and government regulations often change the accepted standard in this field. When consideration is being given to use of any drug in the clinical setting, the healthcare provider or reader is responsible for determining FDA status of the drug, reading the package insert, and reviewing prescribing information for the most up-to-date recommendations on dose, precautions, and contraindications, and determining the appropriate usage for the product. This is especially important in the case of drugs that are new or seldom used.

Production Credits
Senior Acquisitions Editor: Alison Hankey
Senior Editorial Assistant: Jessica Acox
Production Director: Amy Rose
Associate Production Editor: Laura Almozara
Senior Marketing Manager: Barb Bartoszek
V.P., Manufacturing and Inventory Control: Therese Connell
Cover Design: Scott Moden
Cover Image: © Ali Mazraie Shadi/ShutterStock, Inc.
Printing and Binding: Malloy, Inc.
Cover Printing: Malloy, Inc.

Library of Congress Cataloging-in-Publication Data
Grossberg, George T.
   Alzheimer's : The latest assessment and treatment strategies / George Grossberg, Sanjeev Kamat. — 1st ed.
       p. ; cm.
   Includes bibliographical references and index.
   ISBN-13: 978-0-7637-6579-8
   ISBN-10: 0-7637-6579-1
      1. Alzheimer's disease.   I. Kamat, Sanjeev M. (Sanjeev Madhav), 1975–   II. Title.
   [DNLM: 1. Alzheimer's Disease—diagnosis.   2. Alzheimer's Disease—therapy.   WT 155 G878ab 2010]
   RC523.G757 2010
   616.8′31—dc22
                                                                                          2009029047
6048

Printed in the United States of America
13 12 11 10 09   10 9 8 7 6 5 4 3 2 1

Contents

Chapter Three: Pharmacotherapy in Alzheimer's Disease 33

Chapter Four: Psychosocial Treatments for Alzheimer's Disease 61

Chapter Five: Ethical, Legal, and Caregiver Issues in Alzheimer's Disease 73

Appendix: Resources for Caregivers and Physicians   85

Glossary   87

References   91

Index   105

Chapter One
General Information About Alzheimer's Disease

This chapter answers the following:

▶ **What Is Alzheimer's Disease?** This section defines the disorder in the context of a more general definition of dementia.

▶ **How Does Alzheimer's Disease Affect Patients' Lives?** This section discusses the various stages of Alzheimer's disease and their increasing effects on patients' and caregivers' lives.

▶ **How Common Is Alzheimer's Disease?** This section covers the epidemiology of Alzheimer's disease in the United States, including the projected increase in numbers of patients in the coming decades.

▶ **What Are the Risk Factors and Potential Protective Factors in Alzheimer's Disease?** This section discusses the known and proposed risk factors for Alzheimer's disease, as well as known and proposed factors that protect against the disease.

Dementia, a deterioration of cognitive functioning primarily seen in the elderly, is a major public health concern in the United States, both because of increasing life expectancy and the growth of the aging population segment. Alzheimer's disease (AD) is the most common cause of dementia among the elderly. The disease progresses in stages, with each stage bringing further decline to the three primary domains of functioning.

dementia—loss of cognitive and intellectual powers without changes in consciousness

1. Cognition
   ▶ Memory loss
   ▶ Confusion
   ▶ Language difficulties
   ▶ Problems with decision-making or problem-solving

2. Behavior
   ▶ Depression
   ▶ Verbal or physical aggression
   ▶ Wandering
   ▶ Sleep problems

3. Capacity for performing *activities of daily living (ADLs)*
   ▶ Ability to pay bills or shop for groceries
   ▶ Ability to perform self-care, such as bathing and toileting

activities of daily living (ADLs)—daily activities one carries out, from basic activities, such as self-care, to more complex activities, such as paying bills or balancing a checkbook

The disease's slow, insidious path progressively robs patients of their personalities and places increasing stress on their loved ones. It also exacts a financial toll on individuals and businesses. It is estimated that the annual cost of caring for an AD patient ranges from $18,500 to upwards of $36,000, depending on the severity of symptoms. The cost to businesses in insurance claims and lost productivity exceeds $60 billion annually.[1]

Currently, there is limited information about the exact etiology of Alzheimer's disease. Research into the disease, however, has identified a number of risk factors such as head trauma, depression, and genetics. Additionally, there are some putative protective factors such as anti-inflammatory drugs, exercise, and diet.

Making an accurate diagnosis and treating Alzheimer's disease is essential, as treatment not only benefits the patient but may also relieve the stress and burden on family members or other caregivers.

Although there is no cure for Alzheimer's disease, different pharmacological and nonpharmacological interventions may delay the progression of the disease, improve or stabilize its symptoms, and decrease caregiver burden.

What Is Alzheimer's Disease?

Dementia, according to the World Health Organization, is a syndrome caused by a disease of the brain and is usually chronic and progressive. There are different types of dementia, the most common of which is dementia of the Alzheimer's type (Alzheimer's disease).

Alzheimer's disease is a progressive, degenerative brain disorder, clinically defined by a gradual decline in both memory and impairment of at least one other area of higher intellectual function. Such impairments may include *aphasia*, *apraxia*, *agnosia*, or disturbances in *executive functioning*. These changes become severe enough to affect basic daily functioning.[2]

Progressive dementia associated with the abnormal accumulation of *amyloid* protein plaques in the brain is characteristic of the disease. Other distinctive characteristics of Alzheimer's disease include:

► *Neuritic plaques*—degenerate axons and dendrites surrounding an amyloid core

► *Neurofibrillary tangles* (NFTs)—twisted fibers inside the neurons' cell bodies

aphasia—the inability (or impaired ability) to communicate through spoken, written, or sign language; aphasia can refer to the inability to produce such communication or to comprehend it

apraxia—(1) the inability to carry out voluntary movements despite intact muscle control; or (2) the inability to use a familiar object despite being able to recognize the object and its intended function

agnosia—the inability to recognize sensory cues (sights, sounds, etc.) despite normal intelligence and normal functioning of sensory organs (eyes, ears, etc.)

executive functioning—brain functions that allow a person to plan, organize, and carry out goal-oriented behaviors

amyloid—a group of complex proteins that share certain laboratory characteristics and form sheets deposited in various tissues under disease conditions

neuritic plaques—deposits of amyloid in the gray substance of the brain that are associated with destruction of brain structures

neurofibrillary tangles—accumulation of protein fibers twisted within neurons

▶ Loss of neurons

▶ *Amyloid angiopathy*—the presence of amyloid deposits in the brain's small blood vessels

amyloid angiopathy—amyloid deposits in the brain's blood vessels

How Does Alzheimer's Disease Affect Patients' Lives?

The effects of AD on patients and their families vary by the stage of the disease, becoming more pronounced and difficult to manage as the disease progresses. The rate of progression of the disease is different for each patient, and not all patients display every symptom at every stage.

Case Presentation: Mr. J. B.

Mr. J. B., a 69-year-old former police officer, sought an appointment with his physician, wishing, as he put it, "to get my wife off my back." His medical history includes a father who died of Alzheimer's disease. Once retired, Mr. J. B. enjoyed a sedentary lifestyle with the exception of an annual fishing trip he takes with his younger brother. He tells his doctor:

Lately, I have been having problems remembering where I keep my wallet, and I keep misplacing my glasses. I guess this is the price you pay for getting old. I am a little embarrassed to admit that for some time now I haven't been able to use a toothbrush in the mornings—my wife has to help me out with that. You know, I don't think she is faithful to me anymore. I believe she is having an affair with someone. She also tells me that our rent and utility bills are long overdue. I know I have been having trouble doing my finances correctly for a while now, but I think she and her new man are stealing money from me and trying to cover it up.

Stages of Alzheimer's Disease

AD progresses through mild, moderate, and severe stages. The possible symptoms associated with each stage are described as follows.

Mild AD

At this stage, there is some memory loss affecting recall of recent events, which may interfere with the patient's daily activities at home and at work. The patient may show poor judgment in complicated and unfamiliar situations and may have difficulty doing complex tasks such as paying bills or balancing a checkbook. Attention is poor, and a simple test, such as subtracting 7's from 100, will cause the patient difficulty.[3] Depression often occurs at this stage.[4-6]

Moderate AD

Memory loss is more marked at this stage. The patient will probably remember only major events or facts such as the names of loved ones or the patient's own occupation, if employed. There is disorientation to time and place; patients will have difficulty remembering the day of the week, for instance, and may have trouble finding their way even in familiar streets and neighborhoods. Sleep problems are common at this stage and include insomnia and multiple awakenings during the night. Difficulty in speech occurs, with difficulties potentially manifesting as either a decrease in quantity of speech or the repetition of multiple words. Restlessness (especially wandering) often occurs at this stage.[4-6] Patients may also exhibit paranoid or delusional thinking, as well as hallucinations.

Severe AD

Agnosia and apraxia manifest at this stage. Patients may not recognize an object upon visual presentation, even though they may describe its shape and other characteristics. They may not recognize sounds, may have difficulty perceiving objects through touch, and may show an inability to make proper movements in response to verbal commands. Patients have both urinary and fecal incontinence at this stage and need full assistance with activities of daily living, such as bathing and toileting. Physical and verbal aggression and agitation may be present, demonstrated through behaviors such as screaming. Gait abnormalities are also evident. Patients will require assistance with devices such as walkers, and in the final stages of AD, patients may be bedridden.[4-6]

Table 1.1 identifies common features of Alzheimer's disease.

> **Case Presentation: Mr. J. B.**
> Mr. J. B.'s inability to keep his finances in order is in line with mild AD. However, his inability to brush his teeth and his paranoid ideations regarding his wife's "affair" are indicative of a disease that has progressed to the moderate stage. Further evaluation will probably show disorientation to time and place and a recent history of sleep abnormalities, consistent with moderate AD.

Table 1.1   Differentiating Stages of AD by Domain

Domain	Mild AD	Moderate AD	Severe AD
Cognition	• Deficits in recall of recent events and personal details • Worsening ability to concentrate • Evident cognitive decline	• Worsening language skills • Worsening recall of important aspects of one's life such as one's past occupation	• Inability to recognize familiar people such as a spouse or child • Loss of language skills and inability to verbalize needs and emotions
ADL	• Increasing inability to perform instrumental ADLs, including handling of personal finances or planning important events	• Increasing inability to perform basic activities such as eating and toileting without assistance • Increasing inability to perform activities such as dressing and grooming, even with assistance	• Increasing inability to perform basic activities such as eating and toileting without assistance • Increasing inability to perform activities such as dressing and grooming, even with assistance
Behavior	• Decreasing motivation and initiative • Decreasing enthusiasm • Depression and withdrawal	• Increasing agitation, restlessness, and aggression • Increase in paranoid behavior • Increasing hallucinations and delusions • Wandering away from home or nursing facility	• Screaming or shouting even when not in distress • Extreme agitation when assistance is offered or rendered

How Common Is Alzheimer's Disease?

In the year 2000, there were an estimated 4.5 million persons with AD in the United States.[7] By 2007, the number had grown to over 5 million.[8] By 2050, this number will increase by almost threefold to 13.5 million. During this time, and owing to the rapid growth of the oldest age groups in the U.S. population, the number of affected persons who are 85 years and older will more than quadruple to 8 million. The number of affected persons who are 75 to 84 years old will double to 4.8 million, while the number of those who are 65 to 74 years old will remain fairly constant at 0.3 to 0.5 million.[7,9,10]

Surveys done among elderly community residents show that an estimated 5–10% of persons who are 65 years of age or older suffer from AD. Among persons older than 85 years, an estimated 40–50% (or more) suffer from AD.[11]

What Are the Risk Factors and Potential Protective Factors in Alzheimer's Disease?

We currently know more about risk factors for AD than we do about what might protect us from the disease. Only one factor—the presence of the APOE2 *allele* of the gene-encoding *apolipoprotein E*—is known to protect against AD, though several other factors show strong evidence of protection. The following discussion lists known and suggested risk and protective factors and the evidence that supports each.

allele—a form of a gene; for example, the gene for eye color has an allele for blue eyes and an allele for brown eyes

apolipoprotein E (APOE)—a serum protein important in cholesterol transport; persons with the APOE4 allele are at a higher risk for developing AD, while those with the APOE2 allele seem more protected against the disease

Risk Factors

1. *Age:* Increasing age is the greatest risk factor for Alzheimer's disease. As mentioned previously, an estimated 50% or more of those people over 85 years of age suffer from Alzheimer's disease.[12]

2. *Family History:* However rare, inherited forms of Alzheimer's disease can strike individuals even in their 30s and 40s.[12,13] Familial AD, an uncommon type of AD, is characterized by the early onset of the disease (usually at 35 to 60 years of age) with early neuropathological alterations, including amyloid-β (Aβ) deposits.

3. *Vascular Risk Factors:* The following vascular risk factors may increase a person's risk of developing AD:[14]

   ▶ Uncontrolled high blood pressure

   ▶ Diabetes mellitus

   ▶ Smoking

   ▶ Obesity

   ▶ Lack of exercise

4. *Gender:* Women have a slightly greater risk of developing dementia of the Alzheimer's type than men.[15] It is unknown at this time whether this increased risk is due to the loss of the protective effects of estrogen or the fact that women, on average, live longer than men.

5. *Genetic Factors:* Studies have identified three "causative" AD genes for early-onset familial AD (FAD). These are genes in which a mutation is sufficient to cause clinical AD. In addition, one "susceptibility" gene that affects risk and age of onset of AD has been identified.[16] The three causative genes are the amyloid precursor protein (APP) gene on chromosome 21, the presenilin-1 gene on chromosome 14, and the presenilin-2 gene on

chromosome 1. The susceptibility gene is the APOE gene on chromosome 19.

In one study of 42 families with late onset of the disease, the risk for AD increased from 20% to 90%, and the mean age at onset decreased from 84 to 68 years as the number of APOE ε4 alleles increased. Thus, the APOE ε4 allele dose is a major risk factor for late-onset Alzheimer's disease.[17]

A recent study that looked at over 6000 participants from diverse ethnic backgrounds found that variations in the gene SORL1 are associated with late-onset AD. These variations caused an underexpression of SORL1. It is unknown at this time what causes these variations, but an environmental influence is a possibility. The gene suppression resulting from these gene variants diverts APP recycling into an Aβ peptide-producing pathway, which leads to AD.[18]

6. *Down Syndrome*: The presence of Down syndrome is a risk factor for the development of AD. Virtually all individuals with Down syndrome who are over the age of 40 years eventually develop AD and show the characteristic pathological brain changes of Alzheimer's disease at autopsy.[19]

7. *Head Trauma*: Head trauma, especially with loss of consciousness, may be a risk factor for AD. The magnitude of the risk is proportional to the severity of the trauma and is heightened among first-degree relatives of AD patients.[20] Recent research has identified an enzyme, beta-site APP-cleaving enzyme (BACE), which is involved in the production of the Aβ protein associated with AD. Brain injury triggers a series of events in the brain that increase BACE levels, potentially leading to the development of AD.

8. *Metals*: There were early reports that a high concentration of aluminum in drinking water may be a risk factor for Alzheimer's disease, but these reports have not been validated.[21] The current focus is on other heavy metals such as zinc. Epidemiologic evidence for an association between exposure to heavy metals and other environmental agents and AD is not conclusive, although there are theories that there may be causal links, which necessitate more research.

9. *Depression*: Some studies suggest that late-life depression with cognitive changes is a risk factor for the later development of AD.[22] Furthermore, depression may exacerbate AD symptoms and disease progression.

homocysteine—an amino acid that is toxic to the body

10. *Lack of Formal Education*: Not exercising the neurons over a lifetime may be a risk factor.[23]

11. *Elevated Homocysteine Levels*: Some studies have shown that elevated total plasma homocysteine levels are a risk factor for the development of AD.[24]

Protective Factors

1. *APOE2 Genotype*: APOE2 is known to impart protection against developing AD, and patients with the disease who carry at least one E2 allele are likely to develop symptoms of AD only later in life.[25]

2. *Anti-inflammatory Drugs*: One hypothesis holds that brain inflammation is a cause of neuronal injury in AD. Data have shown that anti-inflammatory drugs may act as protective agents.[26]

statins—cholesterol-lowering drugs that are hypothesized to protect against AD

3. *Statins*: At present, there is no good evidence to recommend statins for reducing the risk of Alzheimer's disease.[27] However, ongoing clinical trials are studying statins and the progression of AD. Results of these trials should allow for definitive recommendations concerning the use of statins in the treatment of AD.

4. *Alcohol*: It appears that moderate alcohol consumption lowers the relative risk of developing Alzheimer's dementia.[28] It is unclear whether this is a benefit of the alcohol itself or of other constituents specific to wine, such as polyphenols. The specific antioxidant properties of polyphenols in wine may be particularly important in preventing Alzheimer's disease. Daily consumption of wine is associated with a lower risk of AD.[29]

5. *Education and Intellect*: Some data suggest that increased educational and occupational attainment may reduce the risk of, or delay the onset of, AD, perhaps by increasing cognitive reserves.[30]

6. *Exercise—Physical and Mental*: Epidemiological studies have shown that frequent participation in cognitively stimulating activities, such as reading a newspaper, is associated with reduced risk of AD.[31]

A 2001 study of over 9000 randomly selected participants found that engaging in high levels of regular physical activity is associated with a reduced risk of Alzheimer's disease. In this study, a high level of physical activity corresponded to exercising three or more times per week, at an activity level greater than walking.[32]

Research published in 2003 that related aerobic fitness to loss of brain tissue may help shed light on the connection between physical activity and reduced risk of AD. The study found that the area of the brain most susceptible to *ischemic damage* (the *hippocampus*), which is also one of the earliest areas of the brain to be affected by Alzheimer's disease, suffered less tissue loss in older persons who were more physically fit.[33]

Another 2003 study examined whether there was a lower risk of dementia in patients who participated in leisure activities. This community study looked at 469 people without dementia, all older than 75 years of age. Participants were followed over a median period of 5 years. The study showed that increased participation in leisure activities (i.e., reading, playing board games, playing musical instruments, and dancing) was associated with a reduced risk of Alzheimer's disease.[34]

Burns et al. did a study to examine the correlation of cardiorespiratory fitness with brain *atrophy* and cognition in patients with early stage Alzheimer's disease. The study showed less brain atrophy in individuals with early stage AD who performed well during a treadmill test than in those who were less fit. Since the study was cross-sectional at a single point in time, it was premature to conclude that increased fitness inhibits brain atrophy.[35] In a 1-year randomized, controlled trial done involving 134 ambulatory patients with mild to severe AD in five nursing homes, it was found that an exercise program led to significantly slower decline in activities of daily living score in these patients than routine medical care.[36]

7. *Mediterranean Diet*: Evidence shows that a Mediterranean diet lowers the risk of cardiovascular disease and several forms of cancer. Studies are now showing that a Mediterranean diet may also reduce the risk of AD.[37] Adherence to the entire diet is important—simply consuming certain components of the diet in isolation is not sufficient.

   The Mediterranean diet may decrease oxidative stress and inflammation in the body; it may also lower vascular risks such as hypertension and diabetes. These benefits may combine to help lower the risk of AD.

8. *Omega-3 Fatty Acids*: There is some new evidence that supplementation of the diet with omega-3 fatty acids may reduce the risk of developing Alzheimer's disease.[38] However, a recent placebo-controlled study of omega-3 fatty acids in the treatment of AD showed limited benefits, except for a possible cognitive benefit among patients with very mild dementia. Another recent study, the Three-City cohort study in France, showed reduced risk of AD with increased consumption of omega-3 fatty acids, along with fish and fruits and vegetables, particularly for those who do not carry the APOE4 allele.

ischemic damage—damage to a part of the body resulting from inadequate blood supply

hippocampus—the brain's memory center; it stores and consolidates memories

atrophy—wasting away

omega-3 fatty acids—fatty acids important for maintaining a healthy body and theorized to be protective against AD; omega-3 fatty acids must be obtained through diet, as the body cannot manufacture them

Table 1.2   Summary of Risk Factors and Protective Factors in Alzheimer's Disease

	Confirmed	Strong Evidence	Some Evidence (More Studies Needed)	Theoretical
Risk Factors	• Age • Family history • Genetic factors • Down syndrome • Gender	• Vascular risk factors	• Head trauma • Depression • Elevated homocysteine levels	• Heavy metals • Lack of education
Protective Factors	• Genetic factors (APOE2)	• Moderate alcohol consumption • Exercise—physical and mental	• Mediterranean diet • Omega-3 fatty acids • Increased educational and occupational attainment	• Anti-inflammatory drugs • Statins

Case Presentation: Mr. J. B.

Mr. J. B.'s risk factors include:

▶ A family history of AD

▶ His age—Up to 10% of people over 65 years develop AD.

▶ His sedentary lifestyle—Lack of exercise is a risk factor for AD; it also affects vascular health, another risk factor for AD.

Table 1.2 summarizes risk and protective factors in AD.

Chapter Summary

Alzheimer's disease is a progressive, degenerative brain disorder. It causes worsening deficits in areas of cognition (including executive functions), behavior, and activities of daily living. The disease exacts an emotional, financial, and physical toll on the families it affects. The number of people diagnosed with AD is projected to triple by the year 2050.

A number of factors are known to increase the risk of developing Alzheimer's disease. These factors include increasing age, family history, presence of the APOE4 allele, and female gender. Other possible risk factors, for which there is strong evidence, include vascular risk factors such as obesity, uncontrolled high blood pressure, and smoking.

Much less is known about factors that protect people from AD. Presence of the APOE2 allele is the only confirmed protective factor at this time. Other hypothesized protective factors include mental and physical exercise, moderate alcohol consumption, and adherence to a Mediterranean diet.

Chapter Two
Diagnosing and Assessing Alzheimer's Disease

This chapter answers the following:

▶ **What Are the Typical Presenting Features in Patients With Alzheimer's Disease?** This section reviews the typical presentation of patients with Alzheimer's disease.

▶ **What Are the Criteria for Diagnosing Alzheimer's Disease?** This section presents the accepted criteria from the *DSM-IV-TR* and the NINCDS-ADRDA for diagnosing Alzheimer's disease.

▶ **What Tools Are Available for Clinical Assessment of Alzheimer's Disease?** This section offers direction on conducting clinical interviews and using assessment tools. It also discusses some important laboratory findings, radiological findings, and neuropsychological findings in patients with Alzheimer's disease.

▶ **What Differentiates Alzheimer's Disease From Normal Aging and From Other Disorders?** This section reviews various disorders that may be difficult to distinguish from Alzheimer's disease. It also helps to distinguish Alzheimer's disease from the normal aging process.

Assessing Alzheimer's disease involves identifying the patient's range of symptoms in areas of impaired cognition, activities of daily living, and behavior. The different stages of Alzheimer's disease have been described in Chapter 1. Although memory is an important aspect of cognition, assessing impairment in other areas, such as language and executive function, is necessary as well.

In addition to the *Diagnostic and Statistical Manual of Mental Disorders, Fourth Edition, Text Revision* (DSM-IV-TR) diagnostic criteria, the common diagnostic criteria for AD are those published by the National Institute of Neurological and Communicative Disorders and Stroke, in collaboration with the Alzheimer's Disease and Related Disorders Association (the NINCDS-ADRDA criteria).[39]

DSM-IV-TR—Diagnostic and Statistical Manual of Mental Disorders, Fourth Edition, Text Revision; the standard text setting out the criteria for diagnosing mental disorders

What Are the Typical Presenting Features in Patients With Alzheimer's Disease?

In Alzheimer's disease, there are deficits in three domains: cognition, activities of daily living, and behavior. As a result, symptoms are present in each of these three domains. The presentation of symptoms in each domain varies among patients.

Case Presentation: Ms. L. S.

Ms. L. S. is brought to her internist's office by her daughter, who is deeply concerned about her mother's deteriorating cognitive and functional performance. This patient is a 79-year-old widow who has been living independently since her husband's death 6 years ago. When asked by the nurse whether she is experiencing any particular problems, she replies:

My doctor called me last week and said that I had missed the last three appointments I scheduled. I was amazed at how this had happened—I'm normally so organized. Even worse, when I saw the doctor just now in the hallway, I didn't remember ever seeing him before.

At home, my children keep telling me that I make them repeat what they tell me over and over again. I also haven't been able to prepare my meals for several months now, something I had no trouble with at any other time in my life.

Cognition

Deficits in memory and at least one other area of intellectual function, such as language or executive functioning, occur in Alzheimer's disease.

Memory: Short-term memory loss is most pronounced, and an insidious decline in memory function is a classic symptom occurring in probable dementia of the Alzheimer's type. Common symptoms are forgetting where objects are kept, misplacing objects, difficulty remembering names of friends and acquaintances, and difficulty remembering appointments. Later, intermediate and remote memories become impaired, and symptoms may include the inability to recognize familiar faces such as those of family members.

Language Disturbance: Patients may have difficulty finding the right words, naming objects, and repeating simple or complicated phrases. Language disturbances in the form of aphasia can occur. Patients may have trouble understanding words or have trouble speaking fluently. They may use incorrect or meaningless words while speaking. Language disturbances can also occur in the form of the patient being unable to read and write sentences correctly.

Agnosia and Apraxia: Agnosia is the failure to recognize or identify objects despite intact sensory function. Apraxia is an impaired ability to carry out motor activities despite intact motor function. Both apraxia and agnosia can occur in AD. Patients may have trouble in correctly using a toothbrush to brush their teeth, using scissors to cut paper, or copying or drawing figures. They may have difficulty recognizing objects such as a watch or identifying sounds such as laughter or crying.

Executive Functioning: Problems with executive functioning can lead to symptoms such as difficulty with abstract thinking or planning. Executive functioning deficits also lead to difficulties in problem-solving, decision-making, and organizing.

Activities of Daily Living

Early in the course of AD, more sophisticated activities of daily living (known as instrumental activities of daily living, or IADLs) are lost. These include financial decision-making, cooking, or keeping an appointment book. In later stages, more fundamental activities of daily living, such as bathing, dressing, and hygiene, may be affected.

Behavior

In Alzheimer's disease, cognitive, psychological, and behavioral impairments usually go hand in hand. Psychological and behavioral symptoms include depression, anxiety, irritability, sleep disturbance, psychosis, and agitation.[3] Timing of the appearance of these symptoms is characteristic of the disease's progression. Depression usually occurs up to several years *before* diagnosis. Psychosis may occur around the time of diagnosis, while agitation generally occurs late after diagnosis.[40]

Depression: Rates of clinically significant depression vary from 9% to 60% in patients with Alzheimer's disease. In 2002, separate criteria for depression of the Alzheimer's type were proposed,[41] and these are now widely accepted and validated.

Compared with major depressive disorder (MDD), only three symptoms (rather than five) need to be present during the same 2-week period for diagnosis of Alzheimer's-related depression. One of the symptoms must be either (1) depressed mood or decreased positive affect or (2) decreased pleasure in response to social contacts and usual activities. It is important to keep in mind that depression can occur during any stage of AD and can trigger a more rapid decline in the patient's overall condition. Recognition and treatment of depression can result in functional improvement and disease stabilization.

Psychosis: Psychotic symptoms of both delusions and hallucinations can occur in patients with Alzheimer's disease.[42] The person with AD might have paranoid or persecutory delusions.

For example, the patient may accuse his or her spouse of theft or of having an affair. The patient may talk to people who are not visible to the observer or describe things not seen by the observer.

Agitation: Agitation is common during the course of Alzheimer's disease.[43] It can take the form of physical or verbal aggression, pacing, or wandering.[44] Physical aggression can be in the form of hitting or scratching. Verbal aggression can manifest as outbursts of screaming or cursing or as temper tantrums.

Sleep Abnormalities: Sleep abnormalities increase as Alzheimer's disease progresses.[45] Frequent sleep abnormalities include sleeping more than usual, early morning awakenings, and nighttime awakenings. Caregivers are most distressed with patients who have frequent nighttime awakenings or day/night confusion.

Anxiety: Anxiety symptoms are common in patients with AD.[46] They have been found to correlate with ADL impairment and disturbances such as wandering, hallucinations, and verbal aggression. *Comorbid* depression is often present. Anxiety symptoms seen in AD patients may accompany tension, fears, insomnia, and physical complaints such as pain.[47]

comorbid—a disease or condition occurring at the same time as another disease or condition but unrelated to it

Table 2.1 presents a summary of cognitive, activity-related, and behavioral deficits in AD.

What Are the Criteria for Diagnosing Alzheimer's Disease?

Two sets of criteria are commonly used to diagnose Alzheimer's disease. They are the *Diagnostic and Statistical Manual of Mental Disorders, Fourth Edition, Text Revision* (*DSM-IV-TR*) criteria [48] and the National Institute of Neurological and Communicative Disorders and Stroke—Alzheimer's Disease and Related Disorder Association (NINCDS-ADRDA) criteria.[39]

Both sets of criteria require:

- ▶ Deficits in two or more areas of cognition
- ▶ Progressive decline in the affected areas of cognition
- ▶ Exclusion of other brain and systemic diseases that could cause these cognitive deficits

These published criteria are presented in Tables 2.2 and 2.3.

The diagnosis of probable AD is given to a living patient when there is clinical evidence of AD, but no histopathological examination of brain tissue is done.

Table 2.1   Summary of Deficits in Alzheimer's Disease

Deficits in Cognition
- **Memory**
  - Short-term memory loss (usually an initial sign)
    - Misplacing objects
    - Forgetting names of acquaintances
    - Forgetting where objects are kept
  - Long-term memory loss (a later sign)
    - Forgetting names and faces of loved ones
    - Forgetting past occupation(s)
- **Aphasia or Language Disturbance**
  - Inability to understand spoken words
  - Inability to find the correct words to use
  - Inability to read and/or write
  - Using meaningless sounds instead of words
- **Apraxia**
  - Inability to carry out motor activities, despite intact motor function
- **Agnosia**
  - Inability to recognize common objects
  - Inability to recognize common sounds
- **Executive Functioning**
  - Difficulty with problem-solving
  - Difficulty planning and organizing
  - Difficulty with decision-making

Deficits in Activities of Daily Living (ADLs)
- **Difficulties with IADLs (early sign)**
  - Appointment-setting or -keeping
  - Handling finances
  - Handling household chores
- **Difficulties with simple ADLs (later sign)**
  - Personal hygiene
  - Self-care

Deficits in Behavior
- **Depression**
  - Depression that may precede diagnosis by several years
  - Depression whose treatment may improve overall function
- **Psychosis**
  - Delusions
    - Usually paranoid or persecutory
  - Hallucinations
    - Visual hallucinations more common than auditory
- **Agitation**
  - Verbal or physical aggression
  - Wandering
- **Sleep Abnormalities**
  - Nighttime and early-morning awakenings
  - Sleeping more than usual

Table 2.2   *DSM-IV-TR* Criteria for Alzheimer's Disease

A. The development of multiple cognitive deficits manifested by both

   (1) memory impairment (impaired ability to learn new information or to recall previously learned information)

   (2) one (or more) of the following cognitive disturbances:

      (a) aphasia (language disturbance)

      (b) apraxia (impaired ability to carry out motor activities despite intact motor function)

      (c) agnosia (failure to recognize or identify objects despite intact sensory function)

      (d) disturbance in executive functioning (i.e., planning, organizing, sequencing, abstracting)

B. The cognitive deficits in Criteria A1 and A2 each cause significant impairment in social or occupational functioning and represent a significant decline from a previous level of functioning.

C. The course is characterized by gradual onset and continuing decline.

D. The cognitive deficits in Criteria A1 and A2 are not due to any of the following:

   (1) other central nervous system conditions that cause progressive deficits in memory and cognition (i.e., cerebrovascular disease, Parkinson's disease, Huntington's disease, subdural hematoma, normal-pressure hydrocephalus, brain tumor)

   (2) systemic conditions that are known to cause dementia (i.e., hypothyroidism, vitamin B_{12} or folic acid deficiency, niacin deficiency, hypercalcemia, neurosyphilis, HIV infection)

   (3) substance-induced conditions

E. The deficits do not occur exclusively during the course of a delirium.

F. The disturbance is not better accounted for by another Axis I disorder (i.e., Major Depressive Disorder, Schizophrenia).

Code based on presence or absence of a clinically significant behavioral disturbance:

   294.10 **Without Behavioral Disturbance:** if the cognitive disturbance is not accompanied by any clinically significant behavioral disturbance.

   294.11 **With Behavioral Disturbance:** if the cognitive disturbance is accompanied by a clinically significant behavioral disturbance (i.e., wandering, agitation).

Specify subtype:

With Early Onset:	if onset is at age 65 years or below
With Late Onset:	if onset is after age 65 years

Table 2.3   NINCDS-ADRDA Criteria for Alzheimer's Disease

I. Criteria for the clinical diagnosis of PROBABLE Alzheimer's disease:

   1) dementia established by clinical examination and documented by the Mini-Mental Test, Blessed Dementia Scale, or some similar examination, and confirmed by neuropsychological tests;

   2) deficits in two or more areas of cognition;

   3) progressive worsening of memory and other cognitive functions;

   4) no disturbance of consciousness;

   5) onset between ages 40 and 90, most often after age 65; and

   6) absence of systemic disorders or other brain diseases that in and of themselves could account for the progressive deficits in memory and cognition

II. The diagnosis of PROBABLE Alzheimer's disease is supported by:

   1) progressive deterioration of specific cognitive functions such as language (aphasia), motor skills (apraxia), and perceptions (agnosia);

   2) impaired activities of daily living and altered patterns of behavior;

   3) family history of similar disorders, particularly if confirmed neuropathologically; and

   4) laboratory results of

     • normal lumbar puncture as evaluated by standard techniques,

     • normal pattern or nonspecific changes in EEG, such as increased slow-wave activity, and

     • evidence of cerebral *atrophy* on CT with progression documented by serial observation

III. Other clinical features consistent with the diagnosis of PROBABLE Alzheimer's disease, after exclusion of causes of dementia other than Alzheimer's disease, include:

   1) plateaus in the course of progression of the illness;

   2) associated symptoms of depression, insomnia, incontinence, delusions, illusions, hallucinations; catastrophic verbal, emotional, or physical outbursts; sexual disorders; and weight loss;

   3) other neurologic abnormalities in some patients, especially with more advanced disease and including motor signs such as increased muscle tone, myoclonus, or gait disorder;

   4) seizures in advanced disease; and

   5) CT normal for age

IV. Features that make the diagnosis of PROBABLE Alzheimer's disease uncertain or unlikely include:

   1) sudden, apoplectic onset;

   2) focal neurologic findings such as hemiparesis, sensory loss, visual field deficits, and lack of coordination early in the course of the illness; and

   3) seizures or gait disturbances at the onset or very early in the course of the illness

Case Presentation: Ms. L. S.

The problems described by Ms. L. S. point to several deficits:

- ▶ Memory—her inability to remember her doctor's face
- ▶ Executive functioning—her inability to set and keep her doctor's appointments
- ▶ Possible apraxia—her difficulty in making meals

These deficits, if corroborated in a physical and psychological/neuropsychological examination, would satisfy criteria A1 and A2 of the *DSM-IV-TR*, assuming no other underlying cause is revealed. Since her daughter stated that the problems "seem to be getting worse over time," and there is no reported history of delirium or major personality disorders, Ms. L. S. is a likely candidate for a diagnosis of Dementia due to Alzheimer's Disease, Without Behavioral Disturbances (294.10), With Late Onset.

Ms. L. S. also satisfies criteria I (2, 3, 4, 5) and II (1, 2) of the NINCDS-ADRDA diagnosis matrix. As with the *DSM-IV-TR* criteria, more tests are necessary before a diagnosis of probable Alzheimer's disease can be given.

What Tools Are Available for Clinical Assessment of Alzheimer's Disease?

Family and medical histories and the use of assessment tools such as the Mini-Mental State Examination are important for the clinical diagnosis of suspected Alzheimer's disease. The physician should obtain histories from the patient and a reliable informant such as an immediate family member or caregiver.

There are also recommended laboratory tests that help to rule out reversible causes of dementia. Radiological findings and neuropsychological testing can also add to the clinical suspicion of Alzheimer's disease.

Clinical Interview (Medical and Psychiatric History)

A detailed and thorough clinical interview is an essential part of diagnosing and assessing Alzheimer's disease. The patient, as well as an immediate family member and caregiver, should be interviewed.

Important historical questions checking for cognitive complaints are:[49]

- ▶ What is the presenting complaint?
  - ■ Recent memory loss
  - ■ Confusion
  - ■ Geographic disorientation
  - ■ Difficulty with finances
- ▶ When was cognition last normal?
- ▶ What was the pattern of onset (abrupt or gradual)?
- ▶ How fast is the problem progressing?
- ▶ What other cognitive changes have occurred?
- ▶ Have there been personality, behavior, or mood changes?

During the interview, it is important to ask questions regarding a history of memory impairment, executive functioning impairment, and focal motor or sensory neurological symptoms. These questions should probe especially for agnosia, apraxia, and aphasia. Memory impairment would be indicated by history such as frequent repetitions, frequently misplacing objects, and difficulty remembering recent events. Executive functioning impairment would be indicated by history, such as impaired driving skills, or decreased ability to solve problems or make decisions. A list of all medications the patient is currently taking is important and should include any over-the-counter medications and herbal and botanical supplements. The interviewer should also note any history of alcohol use; behavioral and psychological symptoms such as paranoia, agitation, or depressive symptoms; difficulty in activities of daily living; and family history of a similar illness. Lastly, a mental status examination and a complete medical examination, including a neurological examination, should be done.

Assessment Tools

The following tools can be used to assist in the process of determining a diagnosis of probable AD.

1. *Folstein Mini-Mental State Examination (MMSE):*[3]
   The MMSE is a tool that can be used to assess mental status. It is regularly done as part of the assessment of patients with various types of dementia, including Alzheimer's disease. It consists of 11 questions that assess five areas of cognitive functions: orientation, registration, attention and calculation, recall, and language. Out of a maximum score of 30, scores 19–24 indicate mild impairment, scores 10–18 indicate moderate impairment, and scores 0–9 indicate severe impairment.[3] The test is often used as a screening instrument to document the magnitude of cognitive

capacity and impairment. There is typically a deterioration of 3–5 points per year in AD. The MMSE takes 5–7 minutes to administer and is practical for routine and repeated use for a quick and accurate assessment of cognitive functioning.

2. *SLUMS*: The Saint Louis University Mental Status (SLUMS) Examination is another tool, like the MMSE, for screening patients with dementia. In a study comparing the two, the SLUMS proved slightly better at detecting patients with mild neurocognitive disorder (MNCD), which tends to progress into AD over several years. Both tests were equally sensitive at detecting dementia. SLUMS is a 30-item questionnaire that tests the patient's performance on major cognitive tasks, including memory (patients must recall a list of five items given earlier in the test), attention (i.e., recall facts from a short story the examiner tells the patient), and executive functions (the clock-drawing test). Scores are interpreted with the patient's educational level in mind. For patients with a high school education, scores 1–20 indicate dementia. For patients with less than a high school education, dementia is indicated by scores 1–19.[50,51]

3. *Geriatric Depression Scale (GDS)*:[52] The GDS is one of the most commonly used self-report measures for rating depression in the elderly. It is available in 15-item and 30-item versions with all items formulated as yes-or-no questions. It is easily administered and has been found to be both specific and sensitive, allowing for an easy way to rule in or rule out the presence of depression in older patients. On the 30-item form, scores 0–9 indicate an absence of significant depressive symptoms, scores 10–19 indicate mild depression, and scores 20–30 reflect severe depression.

    Caution should be used in interpreting these scores, however, as patients may score low due to a lack of insight. Family members may produce artificially high scores, as they may confuse depression with dysphoria and other dementia-related mood changes. A thorough clinical interview is important in assessing level of depression.

4. *Barthel Index*:[53] The Barthel ADL Index is a common assessment of the patient's ADL impairments. The index measures the patient's capacity to carry out activities such as feeding, bathing, dressing, and maintaining bowel and bladder control. The original scoring presents results ranging from 0 to 100 in

increments of 5, with patients who score 100 being fully independent and patients who score less than 60 needing significant physical or supervisory help provided by a live-in caregiver or long-term care.

5. *Global Deterioration Scale (GDS)*: The GDS is a seven stage rating scale that can be used to determine whether a person has cognitive impairments that are consistent with dementia (including Alzheimer's disease). Individuals are rated according to a seven-point scale and a score of 4 or higher is usually considered to be indicative of dementia. Score 1 or first stage is normal, score 2 or second stage is age-associated memory impairment, score 3 or third stage is mild cognitive impairment, score 4 or fourth stage is mild AD, score 5 or fifth stage is moderate AD, score 6 or sixth stage is moderately severe AD and score 7 or seventh stage is severe AD. It is however important to remember that AD affects each person differently and in many cases, the stages will overlap.

6. *Functional Assessment Staging (FAST) Scale*: The FAST scale has seven stages showing the functional loss of capacity of people with Alzheimer's disease. Stage 1 is normal and there is no functional decline; in stage 2, which is normal older adult, there is personal awareness of some functional decline; in stage 3, which is early AD, there are noticeable deficits in demanding job situations; in stage 4, which is mild AD, assistance is required in complicated tasks such as handling finances and planning parties; in stage 5, which is moderate AD, assistance is required in choosing proper attire; in stage 6, which is moderate severe AD, assistance is required in dressing, bathing, and toileting and patients may experience urinary and fecal incontinence; and in stage 7, which is severe AD, there is progressive loss of abilities to walk, sit up, smile and speech ability declines to few intelligible words.

7. *Neuropsychiatric Inventory-Questionnaire (NPI-Q)*: The NPI-Q is a 12-item version of the Neurospsychiatric Inventory (NPI) that is completed by a patient informant. It is useful for assessing behavioral and psychological symptoms of dementia (BPSD) and yields scores of symptom severity and caregiver distress. The 12 domains assessed include sleep, appetite, hallucinations, and depression. The NPI-Q is useful for repeated assessments over time to assess both treatment efficacy and patient functioning.

Laboratory Evaluations

In addition to obtaining a detailed history, performing a comprehensive physical and neurological examination, and utilizing some of the tools mentioned previously, completing the following laboratory tests is also important:[54]

metabolic profile—a series of tests measuring levels of various components of the serum, such as albumin, liver enzymes, and glucose

▶ A complete *metabolic profile*

▶ Complete blood counts with differential

▶ Urine analysis

▶ Thyroid stimulating hormone (TSH) study

▶ If TSH level is abnormal, further studies such as free T_3 and free T_4 screening to help evaluate for hypothyroidism or hyperthyroidism

▶ Serum B_{12} and folate studies

Knowledge of serum B_{12}, folate, and TSH levels helps rule out potentially reversible causes of dementia.

The following additional tests may also be useful:

▶ Homocysteine level: An elevated level of plasma homocysteine is a possible independent risk factor for the development of Alzheimer's disease.[55]

C-reactive protein (CRP) level—a measure of inflammatory processes in the body

▶ *C-reactive protein (CRP) level*: CRP is a measure of acute inflammation. Studies have found CRP in the brain tissue of AD patients, although this protein is not found in the normal brain.[56] In addition, studies found that increased plasma levels of inflammatory proteins (including CRP) are a known risk factor for dementia.[57] Thus, measuring CRP levels is often part of the diagnostic workup for AD.

▶ Chest radiography

▶ Electrocardiography (ECG)

▶ Lipid profile

The rapid plasma reagin test for syphilis, HIV testing, and similar studies should be done when indicated. Older people face an increased risk of HIV/AIDS and other sexually transmitted diseases, as evidenced by the increasing rate of AIDS diagnoses in persons over 50 years. Possible reasons for this increase include:

▶ Lack of familiarity with the risk factors for HIV

▶ The belief that HIV affects only younger people

Radiological Findings

Evaluation should include a brain scan, such as a computed tomography (CT) scan or a magnetic resonance imaging

(MRI) exam, to look for space-occupying lesions, bleeds, strokes and ventricular dilatation, and greater cortical atrophy than expected for the person's age. Findings such as atrophy of the temporal *sulci*, temporal horns, or the third *ventricle* may be seen on a brain MRI in people with AD.[58]

sulci—deep grooves on the surface of the brain

PET (Positron Emission Tomography) Scans: Changes seen on PET scans in patients with AD occur before visible structural changes appear on CT or MRI scans. A recent study looked at diagnostic sensitivity and specificity of PET scans that were done using F-fluorodeoxyglucose in 284 patients undergoing evaluation for dementia.[18] Patients received at least 2 years of follow-up for disease progression or a histopathological diagnosis an average of 2.9 years later. Among patients with neuropathologically based diagnoses, PET identified patients with AD with a sensitivity of 94% and a specificity of 73%. According to the study's authors, a negative PET scan indicated that pathological progression of cognitive impairment during the mean 3-year follow-up was unlikely to occur.[59]

ventricle—one of the four chambers in the brain that produce cerebrospinal fluid

Amyloid Imaging: Currently, an autopsy is necessary to obtain a definite diagnosis for Alzheimer's disease. In 2004, investigators described a new PET tracer termed Pittsburgh Compound-B (PIB), which is an amyloid-imaging tracer. PIB was tested in 16 live patients with mild AD and 9 healthy controls. In the AD group, PIB accumulated in areas of the brain that typically contain large numbers of amyloid deposits in AD, especially the *frontal cortex*. Areas of the brain known to be unaffected by amyloid plaques (such as the subcortical white matter) looked the same in the study and control groups. The results, according to the study's authors, suggest that PIB can provide quantitative information on amyloid deposits in living patients and may be useful for diagnosis and monitoring of Alzheimer's disease.[60]

frontal cortex—also known as the prefrontal lobe or cortex, it is the area of the brain largely responsible for executive functions

Genetic Testing

Though there is strong evidence that the APOE4 allele increases the risk of AD, testing for this gene is not recommended for use in diagnosis because it is not specific. Many elderly people without dementia carry APOE4, and not all AD patients have this allele.[61,62]

Neuropsychological Testing

Neuropsychological testing may be beneficial and indicated to clarify or confirm the diagnosis of probable AD. Neuropsychological testing should address differential diagnoses, including other types of dementia and stroke. Again, a good history from the informant is required.

The neuropsychological evaluation should include coverage of all domains needed to assess cognitive functioning in suspected AD. Effort testing to rule out malingering or "faking bad" is commonly included in a neuropsychological evaluation.

The areas to be assessed include:

1. Estimate of premorbid IQ

   ▶ The National Adult Reading Test (NART), a test that requires patients to read 50 unusual English words aloud, is often used as an estimate of premorbid IQ.

   ▶ Wechsler Test of Adult Reading is another commonly used measure of premorbid IQ. It is co-normed with the frequently used Wechsler Adult Intelligence Scale, Third Edition (WAIS-III), and Wechsler Memory Scale, Third Edition (WMS-III), which may provide useful information about a patient's functioning.

2. Abbreviated intelligence testing

   ▶ In patients with suspected AD, administration of a full IQ test is rarely required and may produce fatigue and frustration in the patient. Instead, an abbreviated form can provide useful information.

   ▶ Selected subtests from the WAIS-III or an abbreviated version, the Wechsler Abbreviated Scale of Intelligence (WASI), can be administered to examine patterns of strengths and weaknesses in the verbal and nonverbal domains.

3. Learning and memory

   ▶ Assessment of a patient's ability to learn new material, including the pattern of consolidation and storage deficit, is important in an AD evaluation.

   ▶ Selected subtests from the WMS-III can be used to assess memory functioning. Commonly used subtests include Logical Memory (both the immediate and delayed portions), which requires recall following the auditory presentation of a short prose story and is considered a measure of verbal memory, and Visual Reproduction (immediate and delayed), which provides an indicator of nonverbal memory.

   ▶ A verbal learning test, such as the Hopkins Verbal Learning Test, Revised (HVLT-R), or the California Verbal Learning Test (CVLT) can provide additional information about verbal learning and memory.

4. Orientation
   ▶ Assessment of the patient's orientation to person, place, time, and situation is included in a thorough examination of a patient with suspected AD. This is included in the MMSE, described previously, but can be repeated as often as necessary.

5. Focused and sustained attention
   ▶ The Verbal Series Attention Test can provide information about a patient's ability to focus and sustain attention.

6. Language
   ▶ Language assessment consists of examining numerous facets of language, including naming, aphasia, and fluency.
      ■ The Boston Naming Test (BNT) provides information on a patient's visual and confrontational ability by asking him or her to name both common and less common objects.
      ■ Two commonly used batteries, the Boston Diagnostic Aphasia Examination, Third Edition (BDAE-3), and the Western Aphasia Battery (WAB) assess comprehensive language ability, including auditory comprehension, repetition, confrontation naming, and fluency. Impaired naming and fluency are not language specific, and inferences regarding aphasia should not be drawn from these scores.
      ■ Verbal fluency is assessed using many different instruments. It is usually assessed by asking the patient to list as many words as possible beginning with a certain letter (usually F, A, or S) or in a certain category (such as animals) in 1 minute. The number of words generated, as well as incorrect responses and repetitions, are examined.

7. Visuospatial/visuoconstructional ability
   ▶ The clock-drawing test is a commonly used test for assessing visuospatial and visuoconstructional abilities.[63] In this test, the patient is asked to draw the face of a clock and then asked to draw the hands to denote a certain time (commonly 11:10). Common errors in Alzheimer's disease include perseveration, counter-clockwise numbering, absence of numbers, and irrelevant spatial arrangement, although these errors are not unique to AD.

▶ The Alzheimer's Disease Assessment Scale (ADAS) includes copying tasks to assess visuospatial ability.

8. Higher motor functioning (praxis)

▶ Fingertip tapping speed, a commonly used neuropsychological test, is not a sufficient test of motor functioning in AD, as fingertip tapping speed does not typically deteriorate during mild and moderate AD.

▶ The Boston Apraxia Examination is useful for assessing various types of apraxia. Common types of motor difficulties in AD include oral–facial apraxia leading to problems with speech and both transitive (object-related) and intransitive (symbolic) limb functioning. Assessment of limb functioning includes asking the patient to pantomime actions in response to commands of transitive (familiar actions with objects such as brushing teeth) and intransitive (symbolic movements without objects, such as the sign for crazy) movements, as well as imitations of the examiner performing both types of actions.

9. Executive functioning

▶ Tests such as Trail Making Test A and B (connecting numbers from 1 to 25 in order, then connecting alternating numbers and letters in order) or the Stroop Color and Word Test can be used to assess executive functioning. However, most of these tests have a timed component, leading to a problem with interpretation, as timed tests that have a motor component are often confounded in the elderly by motor slowing, slowing in visual scanning, arthritis, etc.

▶ A qualitative analysis of executive functioning can be made by observing the process throughout the testing.

10. Functional ability

▶ As already discussed, functional ability can be assessed with various instruments, including the Barthel ADL Index and the Global Deterioration Scale/Functional Assessment Staging (FAST) Scale.

11. Effort testing

▶ Effort testing is required in an assessment of possible AD to rule out invalid data due to exaggeration or lack of effort.

▶ Most effort tests cannot discriminate between dementia and poor effort. However, both the Word

Memory Test, a simple test that most unimpaired individuals pass easily, and the Medical Symptom Validity Test (MSVT) demonstrate specificity in differentiating dementia from poor effort or malingering.

Generally, in neuropsychological assessment, timed tasks with a motor component should be avoided in the elderly because of the difficulty differentiating motor slowness from attention or ability.

Assessing all cognitive domains as outlined is important in patients with probable AD.[64] When using neuropsychological testing to document disease progression, the battery of tests can be repeated at a later stage and the results compared. Neuropsychological tests are useful in differentiating AD from various other types of dementias and other causes of cognitive impairment, as the testing can illustrate patterns of deficits, which can then be compared to typical deficit patterns for each disease. For example, people with vascular dementias will have more pronounced attention deficits than will people with AD.[65]

Diagnostic Workup Summary

Table 2.4 presents a summary of the diagnostic workup.

What Differentiates Alzheimer's Disease From Normal Aging and From Other Disorders?

Memory may gradually decline with increasing age, and it is important to distinguish normal changes in memory from Alzheimer's disease. Often, people who have subjective complaints of memory loss will ask doctors whether they have AD. These people should be assessed carefully so that Alzheimer's disease can be ruled out. It is also important to differentiate Alzheimer's disease from other types of dementia, such as probable *vascular dementia* and *Lewy body dementia*.

Normal Aging

In people who age normally, there is no subjective or objective evidence of a memory deficit.

Subjective Cognitive Impairment

Subjective memory complaints have been associated with an increased risk of subsequent dementia in some, but not all,

vascular dementia—dementia resulting from infarcts in the brain's blood vessels

Lewy body dementia (LBD)—dementia distinguished by early psychosis and movement abnormalities as well as characteristic abnormal appearance of neurons in the brain

---

Table 2.4   Summary of the AD Diagnostic Workup

Compare results to established AD criteria (*DSM-IV-TR* or NINCDS-ADRDA).

Clinical interview with emphasis on:
- Particular areas of deficit (memory, executive functioning, etc.)
- Presence of agnosia, apraxia, or aphasia
- Medication inventory (prescription, OTC, and supplements)
- History of alcohol use
- Presence of psychological/behavioral symptoms

Cognitive/functional assessment:
- MMSE or SLUMS
- Geriatric Depression Scale (GDS)
- Barthel (ADL) Index
- Global Deterioration Scale (GDS) or Functional Assessment Staging (FAST) Scale
- NPI-Q for assessment of BPSD
- Additional neuropsychological testing as indicated for assistance with differential diagnosis, and to clarify the patient's strengths and deficits

Laboratory workup:
- Metabolic profile
- CBC with differential
- Urine analysis
- Serum B_{12} and folate
- TSH level
- Optional but useful:
  - Homocysteine levels
  - CRP
  - Chest radiography
  - ECG
  - Lipid profile
- Brain CT, MRI, or PET

A PET scan is done only if early diagnosis is required or if the treating physician suspects *frontotemporal dementia*.

---

studies. In a large sample of healthy elderly Dutch individuals, subjective memory complaints were significantly associated with the development of dementia over 3-year follow-up.[66]

This association was stronger in those subjects who had both memory complaints and poor memory performance. In an Australian community sample, subjective memory complaints did not appear to predict cognitive change or the development of dementia over nearly 4 years of follow-up, once anxiety and depression symptoms were taken into account.[67]

A recent longitudinal study used a single question to assess memory complaints with an average follow-up of 3.2 years and found that subjective memory complaint was a relatively strong predictor of Alzheimer's disease in older persons in whom cognitive impairment was not yet apparent.[68]

Age-Associated Memory Impairment

People with *age-associated memory impairment* have subjective complaints of a memory deficit, such as problems remembering names or appointments, but there is no objective evidence of such deficit on clinical interview or on neuropsychological tests.[69] The person with age-associated memory impairment may also have problems remembering telephone numbers or performing complex tasks.

age-associated memory impairment—subjective complaints of memory impairments in an older person despite formal evaluations showing no deficits

Unlike people with AD, people with age-associated memory impairment usually forget only parts of an experience and often will later remember things they had forgotten earlier. They are usually able to follow written or spoken instructions and are able to use notes to help them remember information.[70] In Alzheimer's disease, memory impairment usually occurs more quickly than the gradually developed deficit of age-associated memory impairment.

Mild Cognitive Impairment

Mild cognitive impairment (MCI) refers to a clinical condition that falls on the spectrum between impairments of normal aging and AD. In MCI, persons experience memory loss to a greater extent than one would expect for age, yet they do not meet currently accepted criteria for clinically probable AD.[71,72] Also, when compared with AD patients, patients with MCI have normal performance on activities of daily living and normal cognitive functioning aside from the short-term memory impairment.[71,72] Patients with MCI have a 50% conversion rate to AD over a period of 4 years.[73]

mild cognitive impairment (MCI)—abnormal short-term memory loss where cognitive functioning remains intact

Vascular Dementia

The course of deterioration in vascular dementia is usually stepwise, while the course of deterioration in AD is, in most cases, slowly progressive.[74] Compared to AD, memory deficits in vascular dementia occur later in the course of the illness, and gait disturbances and urinary problems occur early.[74] Focal neurological deficits may be present on neurological examination. These may include lower facial weakness, positive *Babinski sign*, sensory deficit, and *dysarthria*, which are all consistent with stroke. There is evidence of cerebrovascular disease (CVD) on brain imaging, including multiple large-

Babinski sign—a reflex elicited by rubbing the bottom of the foot. It can identify disease of the spinal cord and brain and is also a primitive reflex in infants. When nonpathological, it is called the plantar reflex, whereas Babinski sign refers to the pathological form.

dysarthria—slurred speech due to muscle weakness, muscle paralysis, or brain injury vessel infarcts or a single, strategically placed infarct in areas such as the thalamus.

Patients with vascular dementia have an irregular pattern of neuropsychological deficits.[75] They can retrieve memories by responding to a stimulus connected with the memory. Compared with its onset in AD, apathy occurs earlier in vascular dementia. In vascular dementia, patients may also display motor perseveration—constant repetitions of previous motor activity or action.

Patients with vascular dementia display levels of cognitive impairments similar to those with Alzheimer's disease, but they display more severe behavioral problems, including depression and anxiety, than do their AD counterparts.[76]

Lewy Body Dementia (LBD)

Compared with AD patients, patients with probable Lewy body dementia have more fluctuations in their cognition, worse visual/spatial symptoms, and worse attention functions. In patients with LBD, early psychotic symptoms (such as visual hallucinations) are more common.[77] Soft signs of Parkinson disease, such as tremors or gait changes, are usually present at the onset of the disease, whereas memory symptoms may occur later in the course of the disease. This sequence is different from the usual AD progression, where memory deficits occur much earlier than gait abnormalities.[78]

Parkinson Disease Dementia (PDD)

More than 50% of patients with Parkinson disease will develop progressive dementia, usually 8 or more years after disease onset. Patients who develop Parkinson disease later in life are more likely to develop *Parkinson disease dementia*.[79] Neuropsychiatric symptoms in Parkinson dementia are different from those in AD.[80] Hallucinations, especially visual hallucinations, are more common and severe in Parkinson dementia patients, whereas wandering, agitation, disinhibited behavior, irritability, and euphoria are more common and severe in AD patients. Depression and apathy are more common in early Parkinson dementia. In AD, depression and apathy are later manifestations of the disease.

Parkinson disease dementia (PDD)—dementia in patients with Parkinson disease; occurs in over 50% of patients with Parkinson disease

Mixed Dementia

Some patients may have overlapping symptoms of two types of dementia, such as probable AD and vascular dementia, or AD and LBD. They are referred to as having a probable mixed dementia. These patients usually do not fall completely under one dementia diagnosis clinically, but may have features of two different types.

Frontotemporal Dementia

Patients with *frontotemporal dementia* may have symptoms such as:[81]

> ▶ Impulsivity, such as going on sudden, expensive shopping sprees
>
> ▶ Disinhibited behavior, such as swearing without provocation
>
> ▶ Ritualistic preoccupation, such as hoarding old newspapers
>
> ▶ Involuntary repetition of another's speech (echolalia) and perseveration of speech (continuous repetition of one or more words)
>
> ▶ Bizarre preoccupation with a particular part of the body, such as the eyes
>
> ▶ Emotional indifference and lack of empathy, such as showing no emotional response toward a friend whose loved one has died

frontotemporal dementia— dementia affecting the frontal and temporal lobes, causing severe personality changes but few memory deficits

Compared with AD patients, patients with frontotemporal dementia may show early disinhibited behavior, marked personality or behavioral changes, and few deficits of memory and cognition. Brain imaging such as CT scans or MRI reveal more pronounced atrophy in the frontal and anterior temporal lobes of the brain.

Geriatric Depression

A dementia-like syndrome may result from depression in the elderly. Delusions and sleep abnormalities are common in both conditions, but in depression the delusions are usually self-depreciating, and sleep disturbances are more predictable as either initial or terminal insomnia. Symptoms such as guilt and true suicidal ideations are primarily associated with geriatric depression.[82]

Chapter Summary

Patients with Alzheimer's disease may present to the clinician with deficits in the areas of cognition, activities of daily living, and behavior. The earliest noticeable sign is a deficit in short-term memory. However, depression actually may be present first, possibly preceding AD diagnosis by several years.

There are two sets of criteria for diagnosing AD: *DSM-IV-TR* and NINCDS-ADRDA criteria. In addition to using these criteria, a full medical workup including brain imaging should be carried out. Cognitive tests such as the MMSE, SLUMS, and Geriatric Depression Scale should be part of the evaluation. Clinicians may choose to administer neuropsychological tests, such as the Trail Making Test or WAIS-III, if cognitive test results are inconclusive.

Differential diagnosis of AD should take into consideration not only different types of dementia (such as Parkinson, vascular, or Lewy body) but also geriatric depression. The latter tends to cause AD-like symptoms, but enough differences exist between depression and AD to enable an accurate diagnosis.

Identifying Alzheimer's disease early and accurately would theoretically allow intervention that slows, halts, or even prevents disease progression or onset. Early recognition and intervention facilitate optimal care of Alzheimer's patients and delay the morbidity associated with this progressive illness.

Chapter Three
Pharmacotherapy in Alzheimer's Disease

This chapter answers the following:

▶ **What Are the Neuroanatomical and Neurochemical Hallmarks of Alzheimer's Disease?** This section reviews behavioral factors involved in AD, details anatomical and neurochemical features of AD, and discusses how imaging studies have helped define the areas of the brain involved in Alzheimer's disease.

▶ **What Medications Are Available for Stabilization or Improvement of Symptoms in Patients With Alzheimer's Disease?** This section covers medications that can treat or stabilize symptoms of AD and includes a review of treatment strategies and efficacy of medication.

▶ **What Medications Are Used to Treat Behavioral and Psychological Symptoms of Dementia in Patients With Alzheimer's Disease, and What Are Their Efficacies?** This section covers medications for treating BPSD in patients with AD and reviews their efficacies.

▶ **What Alternative Treatments Can Be Used to Treat Patients With Alzheimer's Disease?** This section reviews the alternative treatments that have been tried in AD and discusses which ones can be used to treat patients with the disease.

▶ **What Are the Emerging or Disease-Modifying Treatments for Patients With Alzheimer's Disease?** This section covers some of the promising emerging treatments for patients with AD.

▶ **How Does Comorbidity Affect Pharmacotherapy Choices for Alzheimer's Disease?** This section addresses the effects of comorbid conditions on drug therapy for AD patients.

▶ **How Can AD Be Prevented Through Lifestyle Modifications?** This section addresses modifications in one's lifestyle that are helpful in the prevention of AD.

THE field of Alzheimer's disease research is growing rapidly, and more research is now being done on various genetic factors involved in the disease. In addition to studying possible causes, new research is also focusing on novel drug-delivery mechanisms, drugs that can modify the course of AD, and imaging techniques to help in early diagnosis of AD. Some of these imaging techniques were discussed in Chapter 2. This chapter will review the anatomical and physiological bases of AD, along with current and future pharmacological treatments for the disease and/or its symptoms.

What Are the Neuroanatomical and Neurochemical Hallmarks of Alzheimer's Disease?

Biochemical Factors Related to Alzheimer's Disease

acetylcholine—a neurotransmitter that seems to be heavily involved in processes involving learning and memory; its availability is significantly reduced in AD

With a better understanding of the roles neurotransmitters play in neurological diseases came the ability to treat the symptoms of such diseases. In the case of Alzheimer's disease, two neurotransmitters are of particular interest: *acetylcholine* and *glutamate*.

Acetylcholine

glutamate—the most important excitatory neurotransmitter in the brain

cholinergic—relating to or mimicking the action of acetylcholine

Loss of *cholinergic* neurons, which mimic the actions of acetylcholine, is a known phenomenon in AD.[83] This connection between acetylcholine and AD symptoms led to the development of cholinesterase inhibitors (ChEI), the first class of medications approved by the Food and Drug Administration (FDA) for treating dementia. The common mechanism of action for these inhibitors is an increase in available acetylcholine through the inhibition of the catabolic enzyme acetylcholinesterase and, in some cases, inhibition of butyrylcholinesterase (the plasma-equivalent of acetylcholinesterase). Studies show a significant correlation between acetylcholinesterase inhibition and observed cognitive improvement.[84]

Glutamate

excitotoxicity—excessive exposure to glutamate or overstimulation of glutamate's membrane receptors

NMDA receptor—N-methyl-D-aspartate receptor; glutamate receptor

Glutamate is the most common excitatory neurotransmitter in the brain and is involved in most functions of the central nervous system, including movement, learning, and memory. Excessive exposure to glutamate—i.e., overstimulation of its membrane receptors (a phenomenon known as *excitotoxicity*)— leads to neuronal injury or death. Excitotoxicity, especially as mediated by *N-methyl-D-aspartate (NMDA) receptors*, is theorized to be a contributing factor in AD pathology and progression.

Excitotoxic neuronal cell death is mediated in part by the overactivation of NMDA receptors. The NMDA receptor antagonist memantine blocks only excessive NMDA receptor activity, without disrupting normal NMDA receptor activity.[85]

Specific Brain Areas Involved in Alzheimer's Disease

basal forebrain—a brain structure essential to the production of acetylcholine

amygdala—the brain structure important in emotions and reaction to danger

Cholinergic neurons' cell bodies lie in the *basal forebrain* and innervate the cerebral cortex and related structures (i.e., the hippocampus and *amygdala*). They also appear to play an important role in cognitive functions, especially memory. Thus, important brain structures involved in the disease process include the frontal cortex, *temporal cortex*, *parietal cortex*, hippocampus, and amygdala.

Neuroimaging studies that detect changes in patients with Alzheimer's disease include CT, MRI, PET, and SPECT (single photon emission computed tomography) exams.

Brain CT Scan: Findings on CT scans of patients with Alzheimer's disease include central and cortical atrophy and ventricular enlargement. As the clinical stages of AD progress, the degree of cerebral atrophy increases. Cortical atrophy is apparent at an early stage, but ventricular enlargement becomes pronounced at later stages.[86]

MRI: Brain MRI in patients with AD shows temporal, parietal, and generalized atrophy. Cross-sectional studies of patients with AD compared with controls have shown significant reductions in the volumes of structures such as the amygdala and the hippocampus.[87]

PET and SPECT: PET and SPECT studies in patients with AD show bilateral hypoperfusion or hypometabolism in the parietal and temporal cortices; the somatosensory and visual cortices are spared these injuries.

temporal cortex—also known as the temporal lobe, the part of the brain associated with memories, hearing, and the interpretation of sounds, including spoken language

parietal cortex—also known as the parietal lobe, this area of the brain receives pain and tactile information; it also analyzes the combined information from the various senses (sight, sounds, taste, etc.)

What Medications Are Available for Stabilization or Improvement of Symptoms in Patients With Alzheimer's Disease?

Medications used for improvement or stabilization of symptoms in patients with Alzheimer's disease include four cholinesterase inhibitors and memantine, an NMDA receptor antagonist mentioned previously. Symptom improvement, when present, is noted in cognitive function, activities of daily living, and global outcome. The following sections outline the basic pharmacology, safety, and efficacy of each FDA-approved medication available for treating AD.

Cholinesterase Inhibitors (ChEI)

The cholinesterase inhibitors are:

- ▶ Tacrine (rarely used)—inhibits acetylcholinesterase and butyrylcholinesterase
- ▶ Donepezil—inhibits acetylcholinesterase

- ▶ Rivastigmine—inhibits acetylcholinesterase and butyrylcholinesterase
- ▶ Galantamine—inhibits acetylcholinesterase

Mechanism of Action

Acetylcholinesterase and butyrylcholinesterase break down acetylcholine. Their inhibition by the acetylcholinesterase inhibitors increases the levels of acetylcholine in the brain.

In addition to this mechanism of action, galantamine also enhances the action of acetylcholine on nicotinic receptors via *allosteric modulation*, which enhances a neurotransmitter's signaling by binding to an alternate receptor site.[88,89,92]

allosteric modulation—the regulation of an enzyme or protein by binding a molecule at a site other than the protein's active site

Case Presentation: Mrs. C. C.

Mrs. C. C. is 63 years old. She recently received a diagnosis of mild AD and was prescribed a cholinesterase inhibitor. She is now at her target dose of the medication and says:

> *I was taken to the psychiatrist by my husband because of my forgetfulness. The doctor said that I had what they call "probable mild Alzheimer's disease." He gave me some medicine that he said might help. I took it only because I did not want to disappoint and displease my husband. However, I must say that after being on this medicine for almost 6 weeks, I can concentrate better while reading a book and my memory has improved so much that I can remember conversations I had with people earlier in the week. My motivation and interest in things I liked doing in the past also improved, and I was able to pay our utility bills on time this month, something I've neglected for quite a while now.*

Tacrine (Cognex)

Tacrine was the first ChEI to be approved by the FDA (in 1993) for the symptomatic treatment of patients with *mild to moderate* Alzheimer's disease. Because of the association of tacrine with hepatotoxicity, however, it requires baseline and multiple follow-up monitoring of liver function tests, and therefore it is rarely used.[108]

Tacrine must be given four times a day and can interact with medications metabolized by the P450, 1A2 isoenzyme system.

Donepezil (Aricept)

Donepezil was approved for the symptomatic treatment of patients with *mild to moderate* Alzheimer's disease in 1996. The

FDA also approved donepezil for the symptomatic treatment of patients with *severe* Alzheimer's disease in October 2006.

It shows a relative bioavailability of 100% after absorption and reaches peak plasma concentrations in 3 to 4 hours.[88] Consumption of food and time of administration do not affect the drug's absorption.

Donepezil is bound mostly to human plasma proteins and is metabolized by CYP450, 2D6 and 3A4. Inhibitors of the 3A4 isoenzyme can increase the levels of donepezil. Whether there are any consequences to such an increase is unknown at this time.

Rivastigmine (Exelon)

Rivastigmine was the third ChEI to be approved by the FDA in 2000 for the symptomatic treatment of patients with *mild to moderate* Alzheimer's disease. The FDA has since approved it for the treatment of Parkinson dementia as well.

Oral intake of rivastigmine results in an extremely rapid absorption; this drug reaches peak plasma concentrations in 30 to 60 minutes and is the likely cause of the frequent nausea and vomiting side effects. Taking rivastigmine after a full meal delays absorption.

Metabolism of rivastigmine occurs primarily at the site of action, and therefore there are minimal drug-to-drug interactions.[109] Rivastigmine is not metabolized by any of the CYP450 isoenzymes. Its efficacy is strictly dose-related.

The rivastigmine transdermal system, or Exelon patch, was approved by the FDA on July 6, 2007, to treat mild to moderate dementia associated with Alzheimer's and Parkinson disease. The treatment begins with a 4.6-mg, 24-hour Exelon patch. Treatment will be increased to the recommended optimal dose (a 9.5-mg, 24-hour patch) if well tolerated after a minimum of 4 weeks.

The Exelon patch should be placed daily in an area that will not rub against tight clothing and to clean, dry, hairless, intact, healthy skin.

Patients taking Exelon capsules may be asked to stop taking the capsules and to begin using the Exelon patch. Patients taking less than 6 mg of Exelon capsules daily can be switched to the 4.6-mg, 24-hour Exelon patch, and those patients taking between 6 and 12 mg of Exelon capsules daily may be directly switched to the 9.5-mg, 24-hour Exelon patch.[89]

Currently rivastigmine transdermal system is being studied at a higher dose of 15-cm^2 rivastigmine patches in patients with Alzheimer's disease.[91]

Galantamine (Razadyne, Razadyne ER):

The FDA approved the ChEI galantamine in 2001 for the symptomatic treatment of patients with *mild to moderate* Alzheimer's disease.

Galantamine is well absorbed and has absolute oral bioavailability of about 90%; its time to peak concentration is approximately 1 hour.

It is metabolized by cytochrome P450 enzymes, mainly CYP450, 2D6 and 3A4, and is then excreted unchanged in the urine. Inhibitors of both CYP450 pathways cause some increase in oral bioavailability of galantamine.

NMDA Receptor Antagonist: Memantine (Namenda)

As mentioned, memantine preferentially blocks excessive NMDA receptor activity without disrupting normal NMDA receptor activity. It is a noncompetitive, low-affinity receptor blocker. It enters the receptor-associated ion channel when it is excessively open, and most importantly, its off-rate is relatively fast. As a result, it does not accumulate excessively and does not interfere with normal synaptic transmission.[85,93]

Memantine was approved by the FDA in 2003 for the symptomatic treatment of patients with *moderate to severe* Alzheimer's disease.

Memantine is well absorbed after oral administration. Food has no effect on the absorption of memantine, and the drug has a half-life of 60–80 hours.

The CYP450 enzyme system does not play a significant role in the metabolism of memantine, but a reduced target dose is recommended in patients with severe renal impairment. Coadministration of memantine with a ChEI does not affect the pharmacokinetics of either compound.

Recently a 24-week, double-blind, placebo-controlled trial of a once-a-day, slow-release 28-mg dose of memantine formulation was completed in patients with moderate to severe AD who were receiving concurrent, stable treatment with a cholinesterase inhibitor. The results for memantine were statistically significant versus placebo, and this preparation may be available next year.[94]

Case Presentation: Ms. K. S.

Ms. K. S. was transferred to a special care unit within her nursing home because her condition and behavior had worsened considerably. The 77-year-old woman has severe Alzheimer's disease. The physician at the special care unit prescribed memantine in addition to the cholinesterase inhibitor she was already taking. Her son says:

My mother was screaming a lot and cursing a lot and scratching a lot even when we weren't doing anything to her (she was worse when we tried to wash her or do anything that required touching her). She didn't recognize even my brother and me anymore, and she also had problems with wetting herself. Her psychiatrist at the special care unit recently put her on some extra medications. It's been 8 weeks since she started taking them, and I noticed that she does not curse or scratch anymore when the nurses (or I) take care of her, even when we touch her. She does scream sometimes when they give her a bath or brush her hair, but only a little. When my brother and I go to see her, she recognizes us and she smiles a little. Her language is also better—she can say a few words to tell us she needs something. She still requires total assistance with everything, but she doesn't resist it as much as before.

Table 3.1 presents a summary of AD medications with their dosage information and common side effects.

Treatment Recommendations for Patients With Alzheimer's Disease

While there are no universally accepted treatment algorithms as such for Alzheimer's disease, organizations such as The Alzheimer's Association and the National Institutes of Health provide treatment recommendations regarding medications and behavioral interventions. The following algorithm may be used for treating AD, based on severity of symptoms.

- ▶ *Mild AD*: Use any of the four cholinesterase inhibitors.
- ▶ *Moderate AD*: The cholinesterase inhibitors or memantine may be used. A combination of memantine and a cholinesterase inhibitor may also be used.
- ▶ *Severe AD*: Use memantine or donepezil alone, or use a combination of memantine and any cholinesterase inhibitor.

Anticipated Responses to Medication According to AD Stage

Table 3.2 summarizes the responses clinicians can expect when treating patients with the four cholinesterase inhibitors and memantine. These observations are based on the authors' clinical practice.

Table 3.1   Summary of AD Medications With Their Dosages and Side Effects

Medication	Starting Daily Dose (mg/d)	Maximum Recommended Daily Dose (mg/d)	Recommended Administration Schedule	Common Side Effects
Tacrine (rarely used)	40	160	Four times daily	Liver damage causing increase in ALT; nausea, indigestion, vomiting, diarrhea, abdominal pain, skin rash
Donepezil	5	10	Once daily in morning or at bedtime	Nausea, diarrhea, insomnia, vomiting, muscle cramps, fatigue, loss of appetite
Rivastigmine	3	6–12	Twice daily after meals	Nausea, vomiting, loss of appetite, weight loss, diarrhea, heartburn
Rivastigmine, transdermal	4.6 (per 24 h)	9.5 (per 24 h), or 10-cm patch	Once daily	
Galantamine	8	16–24	Twice daily after meals	Nausea, vomiting, diarrhea, weight loss
Galantamine ER	8	16–24	Once daily after a meal	
Memantine	5	20	Twice daily	Dizziness, headaches, constipation, pain, hypertension, somnolence, fatigue

Efficacy of Treatment

All four cholinesterase inhibitors are efficacious in stabilizing or improving cognitive function, activities of daily living, and global outcomes in patients with mild to moderate AD. Memantine in combination with one of the cholinesterase inhibitors is effective in treating patients with moderate to severe AD.[95] (Donepezil is also FDA-approved as a monotherapy in moderate to severe AD.[88]) All four cholinesterase inhibitors can cause low heart rate (bradycardia) or heart block in patients with cardiac conduction abnormalities.

Evidence of efficacy of the ChEIs and memantine is discussed next.

Tacrine (Cognex)

Tacrine has been shown to be efficacious in improving cognitive functions, global outcomes, and activities of daily living in patients with mild to moderate Alzheimer's disease.[96] Because of issues of hepatotoxicity, and because this medication is so rarely used, supporting studies will not be discussed here.

Table 3.2　Representative Responses to Antidementia Therapy by Domain at Various Stages of AD

Domain	Mild AD	Moderate AD	Severe AD
Cognition	• Improved recall of recent events and personal details • Improved ability to concentrate or slowing of cognitive decline	• Improved ability to use appropriate words in spoken sentences • Improved ability to remember important aspects of one's life such as one's past occupation	• Improved ability to recognize familiar persons such as a spouse • Improved ability to use words or sounds when help is needed
ADLs	• Increased ability to perform IADLs such as handling of personal finances and paying bills on time • Improved ability to plan ahead	• Improved ability to perform basic ADLs such as eating and toileting without assistance • Improved ability to perform ADLs such as dressing and grooming with assistance	• Less resistance to ADL care rendered by caregivers or nursing staff in a hospital or nursing home • Less resistance to using a wheelchair or walker
Behavior	• More motivation, initiative, and enthusiasm • Improvement in mood and less withdrawn behavior	• Minimal agitation and almost no aggression • Reduced paranoid behavior and reduced intensity of hallucinations and delusions	• Less screaming or shouting when not in distress • Decreased agitation when getting assistance with ADLs

Note: In many cases, there may not be improvement, but rather stabilization or slowing in the expected rate of decline in cognitive functioning, ADLs, or behavioral symptoms at the various stages of AD.

Donepezil (Aricept)

A recent Cochrane review looked at all unconfounded, double-blind, randomized controlled trials of donepezil[97] in which treatment with donepezil was compared with placebo for patients with mild, moderate, or severe dementia due to Alzheimer's disease. There were a total of 24 trials involving 5796 participants. The trials were mostly 5 to 6 months in duration. Outcome measures included domains of cognitive function, activities of daily living, and behavior. The review concluded that patients treated for periods of 12, 24, or 52 weeks with donepezil experienced benefits in all three outcome measures. A variety of adverse effects were also recorded. The treatment group receiving 10 mg/d experienced more incidents of nausea, vomiting, diarrhea, muscle cramps, dizziness, fatigue, and anorexia than the placebo group, but very few patients discontinued the study as a direct result of drug side effects. Benefits of the 10-mg/d dose were marginally greater than the 5-mg/d dose.

The FDA approved donepezil for severe AD based on results from two 24-week, randomized, placebo-controlled trials that were conducted in Sweden and Japan and involved more than 500 patients.[88,98]

The Swedish study was a 6-month, double-blind, parallel-group, placebo-controlled study in 248 patients with severe Alzheimer's disease (MMSE score 1–10). The patients all lived in assisted-care nursing homes staffed by trained caregivers.[98] The treatment group received oral donepezil at 5 mg/d for 30 days, increased up to 10 mg/d thereafter. As compared with placebo-treated patients, those treated with donepezil had significant improvements in cognitive function from baseline. Patients also showed slower decline in daily functioning from baseline. The incidence of adverse events was comparable between the treatment and placebo groups. Most adverse events were transient and mild or moderate in severity.

The second study was conducted in 325 patients with severe AD living in the community or in assisted-living facilities in Japan. These patients were randomized to donepezil 5 mg/d, 10 mg/d, or placebo. Statistically compared with patients in the placebo group, the patients in the group taking 10 mg/d of donepezil had significantly better scores on tests of cognitive functioning and clinician's impression of change. The 5-mg/d dose of donepezil showed a statistically significant superiority to placebo on tests of cognitive functioning, but not on clinician's impressions of change.[88]

Based on the two studies, the dose recommended for use in patients with severe AD is 10 mg/d. The increase in dose from 5 mg/d to 10 mg/d should occur after 4–6 weeks of treatment to minimize the chances of cholinergic side effects.

Rivastigmine (Exelon)

The efficacy of rivastigmine was established in a number of large, multicenter, randomized, double-blind, placebo-controlled trials lasting 3–6 months. The medication improved cognitive function, global outcome, and activities of daily living in patients with mild to moderate Alzheimer's disease.[99] Results indicating that rivastigmine is particularly effective in patients with rapidly progressive AD are consistent with the possible advantage of inhibiting both acetylcholinesterase and butylcholinesterase.[100]

An open-label, 6-month study evaluated the efficacy and safety of rivastigmine in 382 AD patients. These patients had previously failed donepezil treatment because of tolerance problems, lack of efficacy, or both. Patients receiving rivastigmine treatment showed improvement or stabilization in global function, activities of daily living, and cognition. Rivastigmine was generally well tolerated, with the most common adverse events being nausea and vomiting. The study concluded that rivastigmine treatment appeared to benefit AD patients who did not respond to, or could not tolerate, donepezil.[101]

A 24-week, multicenter, randomized, double-blind, placebo- and active-controlled trial compared the efficacy, safety, and tolerability of the once-daily rivastigmine transdermal patch with conventional twice-daily rivastigmine capsules in patients with moderate Alzheimer's disease.[102] The study was conducted in 21 countries and involved 100 centers and 1195 patients aged 50–85 years. All patients had scores of 10–20 on the MMSE.

There were two patch sizes in the study—a 10-cm patch that provides 9.5 mg over 24 hours (the target dose) and a 20-cm patch that provides 17.4 mg over 24 hours. Both patches had better efficacy than the placebo. The target dose showed similar efficacy to the highest doses of Exelon capsules, but differences in side effects. Only 7.2% of patients on the 10-cm Exelon patch reported nausea compared to 23.1% of patients on 12mg/day Exelon capsules, and 6.2% of patients on the 10-cm Exelon patch reported vomiting compared to 17.% of patients on 12mg/day of Exelon capsules.[90] The 20-cm patch showed even greater improvement on cognitive scores versus capsules than that provided by the 10-cm patch, but patients experienced adverse gastrointestinal events similar in number to those experienced with capsules. Local skin tolerability was good in patches of both sizes. The patch also demonstrated good skin adhesion over 24 hours both in hot weather and in a range of everyday situations such as bathing.[102]

Galantamine (Razadyne, Razadyne ER)

The efficacy and safety of galantamine were assessed in several clinical trials. A 3-month, international, multicenter, randomized, double-blind, placebo-controlled trial looked at 386 patients with mild to moderate Alzheimer's disease. Patients in the treatment arm received final doses of 24 mg/d or 32 mg/d (doses were increased over 4 weeks). Galantamine treatment produced significant changes, compared with placebo, in ADLs, IADLs, and cognitive function. There were no improvements in behavioral symptoms. The medication was well tolerated.[103]

A 5-month, multicenter, placebo-controlled, double-blind trial enrolled 978 patients with mild to moderate AD. The treatment groups received doses of 8 mg/d, 16 mg/d, and 24 mg/d. Patients treated with 16 mg/d or 24 mg/d showed significant improvement in cognition, activities of daily living, and behavior. Galantamine was well tolerated at all doses. Slower dose increase seemed to minimize the number and severity of adverse events.[104]

A review published in January 2006 summarized the data on the clinical effects of galantamine in patients with probable or possible Alzheimer's disease and in patients with mild cognitive impairment (MCI).[105] The review concluded that galantamine improved or maintained patients' performance in three major domains—cognitive function, ADLs, and behavior. There was no statistically significant dose effect. However, the efficacy of doses above 8 mg/d was often statistically significant. The drug's safety profile was similar to that of other cholinesterase inhibitors with respect to gastrointestinal symptoms, and adverse effects appeared to be dose-related. The dose best tolerated was 16 mg/d, and there was no increased efficacy in higher doses. For this reason, the reviewers suggested it might be the optimal starting dose for treatment.

The prolonged-release, once-daily formulation of galantamine at 16–24 mg/d shows a similar efficacy and side effect profile as the equivalent twice-daily regimen.

Memantine (Namenda)

Investigators studied memantine as a monotherapy and as a part of a combination therapy in the treatment of moderate to severe AD.

A multicenter, randomized, double-blind, placebo-controlled trial was conducted in 250 outpatients with moderate to severe AD to assess the efficacy of memantine in this population. The treatment group received memantine at a dose of 20 mg/d for a total of 28 weeks. The treatment group showed significantly less decline on global, functional, and cognitive measures during treatment. Memantine was well tolerated, and adverse events in the treatment group were very similar to those in controls. Notably, more agitation occurred in the placebo group than in the memantine group.[106]

Another study also compared the efficacy and safety of memantine to placebo, but in patients with moderate to severe AD already receiving stable treatment with donepezil. This randomized, double-blind, placebo-controlled clinical trial enrolled 404 patients, of which 322 (78%) completed the trial. The patients all had a diagnosis of moderate to severe AD and MMSE scores of 5–14. Participants were randomized to receive memantine (starting dose 5 mg/d, gradually increased to 20 mg/d, n = 203) or placebo (n = 201) for 24 weeks. The memantine treatment group had significantly better outcomes than did the placebo group on measures of cognition, activities of daily living, global outcome, and behavior. The combination of memantine and donepezil was safe and well tolerated. There were no clinically important differences between the treatment and placebo groups in terms of patient mortality, severe adverse events, electrocardiogram abnormalities, vital signs, urinalysis parameters, or potentially clinically important hematologic or biochemical abnormalities. No significant differences in physical exam results were noted between the groups. Notably, the incidence of diarrhea and fecal incontinence was lower in the memantine/donepezil treatment group, a finding that may reflect the 5-HT3 receptor-blocking effects of memantine.[107]

What Medications Are Used to Treat BPSD in Patients With Alzheimer's Disease, and What Are Their Efficacies?

The possible BPSD in AD were discussed in Chapter 2. Over half of patients with AD have BPSD. Nonpharmacological approaches such as environmental and behavioral interventions should be tried before drug interventions; Chapter 4 discusses these approaches. This chapter describes various pharmacotherapeutic interventions, including typical and atypical (second generation) antipsychotics, anticonvulsants, cholinesterase inhibitors, and memantine. Representative studies documenting the efficacy of these treatments are also discussed.

Atypical Antipsychotics

Although *atypical antipsychotics* are used in the treatment of behavioral and psychological symptoms in patients with AD, there is no FDA approval for this indication, and their use is off-label. At present, atypical antipsychotics have shown modest benefits, but more controlled trials are needed to document their efficacy and safety in this patient population.[110]

atypical antipsychotics—second-generation antipsychotic medications with fewer side effects than first-generation medications

In April 2005, the FDA ordered all atypical antipsychotics to carry a black-box warning in their package inserts, stating:[111]

> Elderly patients with dementia-related psychosis treated with atypical antipsychotic drugs are at an increased risk of death compared to placebo. Analysis of 17 placebo-

controlled trials (modal duration of 10 weeks) in these patients revealed a risk of death in the drug-treated patients of between 1.6 to 1.7 times that seen in placebo-treated patients. Over the course of a typical 10-week controlled trial, the rate of death in drug-treated patients was about 4.5%, compared to a rate of about 2.6% in the placebo group. Although the causes of death were varied, most of the deaths appeared to be either cardio-vascular (i.e., heart failure, sudden death) or infectious (i.e., pneumonia) in nature.

Risperidone

mixed dementia—concurrent symptoms of two or more types of dementia

Patients with AD, vascular dementia, or *mixed dementia* showed an improvement in agitation, aggression, and psychosis when treated with risperidone (mean dose 1 mg/d). A combined analysis of three randomized, placebo-controlled trials showed the medication is well tolerated.[112]

Olanzapine

The efficacy and safety of olanzapine in the treatment of psychosis and/or agitation/aggression were evaluated in 206 patients with AD.[113] Patients were randomized to a placebo arm and fixed-dose arms of 5 mg/d, 10 mg/d, or 15 mg/d of olanzapine. Treatment lasted 6 weeks. Low doses of olanzapine (5 mg/d and 10 mg/d) were significantly superior to placebo in treating agitation/aggression and psychosis associated with AD. The 15-mg/d dose did not show significant benefits compared to placebo. Both low doses were well tolerated.

Quetiapine

One study compared the efficacy, safety, and tolerability of quetiapine to those of placebo in the treatment of agitation associated with dementia.[114] It focused on 333 elderly patients residing in long-term care facilities. This was a 10-week, multicenter, double-blind, fixed-dose trial. Patients were randomized to treatment with quetiapine (100 mg/d or 200 mg/d), or placebo. The 200-mg/d treatment group showed a statistically significant reduction in agitation compared with the 100-mg/d and placebo groups. The 200-mg dose was also well tolerated in the study population.

Aripiprazole

In a multicenter, double-blind, placebo-controlled, outpatient study, 208 patients with Alzheimer's disease and psychosis were randomly assigned to aripiprazole or placebo.[115] The aripiprazole dose was titrated upward to a final dose of 5 mg/d, 10 mg/d, or 15 mg/d according to efficacy and tolerability. Patients were kept on their final doses for 10 weeks. The mean dose of aripiprazole at the end of the study was 10 mg/d. The medication was safe and well tolerated. There was no improvement in psychotic symptoms in the treatment group compared with those in the placebo group on the Neuropsychiatric Inventory (NPI)—Psychosis subscale. However, statistically significantly greater effects in the treatment group showed on the Brief Psychiatric Rating Scale—Core and Psychosis assessments.

Ziprasidone

There are no controlled studies of this medication in patients with BPSD.

> **Case Presentation: Mr. G. B.**
> Mr. G. B. is 82 years old and is living with his son and his son's family. His increasingly confused and erratic behavior led to a diagnosis of moderate Alzheimer's disease. In addition to taking a cholinesterase inhibitor, he has also started taking an atypical antipsychotic medication (prescribed off-label). The doctor explained to members of his family the risks and benefits of this new medication, and they felt the potential benefits outweighed the risks. His son recently told the family physician:
>
> *My father was recently given a diagnosis of "probable moderate Alzheimer's disease." He had been forgetting basic things like my name—that was a real blow! He was also having paranoid thoughts that people were stealing from him, and he kept getting angry day and night. He couldn't do even basic things such as going to the bathroom without help. Since being on medications for 2 months, his memory is a little better—if you tell him the names of people he meets, he can remember them for some time. Also, he is less paranoid and gets agitated only during the nights, not during the day. He can do things better, like going to the bathroom by himself, and he lets me help him brush his teeth. He used to scream at me before when I tried to help—he'd forget who I was and it scared him. I think we were all scared—the medicines made a good difference.*

Typical or Conventional Antipsychotics

Side effects of the typical antipsychotics include tardive dyskinesia (involuntary movement of the face and tongue), parkinsonism (including tremors and rigid movements), akathisia (inability to sit still), constipation, and urinary retention.[116,117]

Antidepressant Medications

A 2005 review of five studies looked at use of antidepressants for the treatment of BPSD.[118,119] All five studies were double-blind, placebo-controlled, randomized trials involving the use of serotonergic antidepressants such as sertraline, fluoxetine, citalopram, and trazodone. Overall, the results showed no statistically significant efficacy for treating BPSD symptoms other than depression. One study of citalopram did show positive effects on agitation.[118]

Benzodiazepines

Benzodiazepines such as lorazepam should be used only if required during treatment of acute symptoms that do not respond to other agents. Benzodiazepines are not preferred in the elderly population because of their side effects of worsening confusion, excessive sedation, and increased risk of falls.

Anticonvulsants

Valproate or Divalproex

Some placebo-controlled clinical trials have suggested that valproate may be useful in the treatment of agitation associated with AD. For example, a randomized, double-blind, placebo-controlled trial in 56 patients with dementia and agitation found that patients receiving divalproex sodium showed a statistically significant reduction in agitation over those receiving placebo.[120]

Other studies do not support this conclusion.[121] A randomized, double-blind, placebo-controlled trial looked at 153 nursing home residents with probable or possible AD and agitation. Participants were randomized to 6-week treatment with divalproex sodium at a target dose of 750 mg/d or placebo, with a mean divalproex dose in the treatment group of 800 mg/d. Change in mean agitation scores did not differ between the treatment and placebo groups.

The mood stabilizer sodium valproate inhibits a kinase likely involved in the abnormal phosphorylation of tau protein in Alzheimer's disease, glycogen synthase kinase 3beta.[122,123]

A multicenter, NIH-sponsored study was recently completed to determine if chronic valproate administration to participants with AD who lack agitation and psychosis at baseline would delay the emergence of agitation and/or psychosis and to determine whether valproate would attenuate clinical progression of illness measured by a reduced rate of cognitive or functional decline. This randomized, placebo-controlled, double-blind, multicenter 26-month trial of valproate at a target dose of 10–12 mg/kg/day in 300 outpatients with mild to moderate AD who lack agitation and psychosis at baseline is completed and awaiting data analysis.[124]

Carbamazepine

Two small trials using carbamazepine yielded contradictory results. A 1998 study yielded positive results in treating BPSD, while a 2001 study found negative results.[125,126] Because of these two trials, along with concerns of hematologic toxicity and problematic drug–drug interactions (especially in the elderly), carbamazepine is generally not recommended for the treatment of BPSD.

Cholinesterase Inhibitors

Cholinesterase inhibitors (ChEI) offer an approach to treating BPSD by addressing the cholinergic deficit that may trigger BPSD development.

Donepezil

Donepezil has shown efficacy in treating behavioral problems in noninstitutionalized patients with moderate to severe AD. Studies in patients with mild to moderate AD yielded conflicting results.[127]

Rivastigmine

Rivastigmine has been shown to improve behavioral disturbances in patients with different types of dementia, but most of the studies cited behavior as a secondary endpoint. The behaviors that showed the most improvement included apathy, anxiety, delusions, and hallucinations.[128]

Galantamine

A study of 978 patients with mild to moderate AD randomly assigned treatment with placebo or galantamine (8 mg/d, 16 mg/d, or 24 mg/d). Behavioral changes in these patients were assessed with the Neuropsychiatric Inventory (NPI). The study's authors found that treatment with galantamine reduced onset of new behavioral disturbances and improved existing behavioral problems.[129]

Memantine

A 2006 publication described the results of a hypothesis-generating, 24-week, double-blind, placebo-controlled trial of memantine treatment. Patients with moderate to severe AD received 20 mg/d of memantine. These patients were already receiving stable donepezil treatment. Significant differences favoring memantine over placebo were observed on the 12-item NPI. Treatment with memantine reduced agitation, aggression, irritability, and appetite abnormalities. Memantine also delayed the emergence of agitation or aggression in patients who did not have these symptoms at the time they enrolled in the study.[130] These findings support conclusions of several other studies, beginning with those of a 2003 study that showed a statistically significant difference in NPI values for agitation or aggression in patients receiving memantine.[106]

Outpatients with moderate to severe AD who received memantine performed better on behavioral measures than those treated with placebo. Post-hoc analyses suggest that memantine treatment was associated with a reduced severity or emergence of specific symptoms, particularly agitation and aggression.[131]

A pooled analysis conducted in people with agitation/aggression or psychosis from three large 6-month, randomized studies in moderately severe to severe AD showed that memantine may be a safe and effective treatment in AD patients with agitation/aggression or psychosis.[132]

What Alternative Treatments Can Be Used to Treat Patients With Alzheimer's Disease?

Estrogen

Clinical trials of treatment with oral, conjugated, equine estrogen showed it is not an effective treatment for AD in postmenopausal women.[133,134] There are also known risks of estrogen therapy such as increased risks of thromboembolism and gynecological cancers. Hence, estrogen is not recommended for the treatment of cognitive or functional deficits attributable to AD.

Omega-3 Fatty Acids

There is evidence that omega-3 fatty acid supplements may delay the progression of Alzheimer's disease.[38] Epidemiological and animal studies have suggested that dietary fish or fish oil rich in omega-3 fatty acids (such as docosahexaenoic acid and eicosapentaenoic acid) may decrease the risk of Alzheimer's disease.

A randomized, double-blind, placebo-controlled clinical trial was conducted to determine the effects of dietary omega-3 fatty acid supplements on cognitive functions in patients with mild to moderate AD.[135] The primary measure of cognitive function was the MMSE. Investigators found a significant reduction in MMSE decline rate in the mild AD group who received omega-3 fatty acids compared with the group who received placebo. Omega-3 fatty acid treatment was safe and well tolerated in the AD population.

An NIH-funded, Phase III clinical trial to determine whether chronic supplementation of docosahexaenoic acid (DHA) slows the progression of cognitive and functional decline in people with mild to moderate Alzheimer's disease was recently completed. In this trial, 402 people with mild to moderate AD were randomized to receive 2 grams of DHA or placebo.[136,137] The results showed that DHA treatment did not slow the rate of change on tests of mental function, global dementia severity status, activities of daily living or behavioral symptoms. However we do not know whether patients at risk for AD who take omega-3 fatty acids, whether omega-3 fatty acids may decrease risk for AD or delay onset of AD in these patients or not.

Vitamin C and Vitamin E

Low concentrations of vitamins C and E (both antioxidants) have been observed in the cerebrospinal fluid (CSF) of AD patients, and supplementing these vitamins may delay the development of the disease. Major targets for oxidation in the brain are lipids and lipoproteins.[138]

Results of a placebo-controlled trial showed that vitamin E supplements of 2000 IU/d slowed disease progression in patients with moderate AD.[139] Investigators also studied 10 patients with AD who received daily supplements of 400 IU vitamin E and 1000 mg vitamin C for 1 month. They compared these patients to 10 patients with AD who received daily doses of 400 IU vitamin E alone.[140] They found that the combination treatment significantly increased the concentrations of both vitamins in plasma and CSF. In addition, abnormally low concentrations of vitamin C returned to normal level following treatment and, as a consequence, the susceptibility of CSF and plasma lipoproteins to in vitro oxidation was significantly decreased. Notably, supplementing with vitamin E alone significantly increased its CSF and plasma concentrations but was unable to decrease the lipoproteins' sensitivity to oxidation. These findings may support the superiority of combined vitamin E and vitamin C supplement treatment over vitamin E supplementation alone in AD. Use of high-dose vitamin E supplements in excess of 400 IU/d is associated with a higher mortality risk and is therefore not recommended.[141]

Mediterranean Diet

The association between a Mediterranean diet and Alzheimer's disease was examined in a study published in 2006. The authors conducted a case-control study involving 1984 patients. Their results showed that a greater adherence to a Mediterranean diet was associated with a significantly lower risk of Alzheimer's disease. Compared with people whose diets scored in the lower third of similarity to the Mediterranean diet, those with diets in the upper third were 69% less likely to have Alzheimer's disease.[37]

The association between the Mediterranean diet and mortality in patients with AD was examined by prospectively following 192 people diagnosed with AD living in the community. They were assessed every 1.5 years. It was found that higher adherence to the Mediterranean diet was associated with lower mortality.[142]

A meta-analysis of prospective cohort studies that analyzed the relation between adherence to the Mediterranean diet and health status revealed that adherence to a Mediterranean diet was associated with a significant reduction in the incidence of Alzheimer's disease.[143]

Recently, higher adherence to the Mediterranean diet was also shown to be associated with a reduced risk of developing mild cognitive impairment and reduced risk of conversion from mild cognitive impairment to AD.[144]

What Are the Emerging or Disease-Modifying Treatments for Patients With Alzheimer's Disease?

Amyloid-β (Aβ) deposition may be the primary culprit in AD, but other putative downstream pathologies may also play a role in AD pathogenesis.[145] These pathologies include:

- The aggregation of phospho-tau in neurofibrillary tangles
- Synaptic and neuronal loss
- Glial and inflammatory responses

The currently available cholinesterase inhibitors and memantine are safe and effective when it comes to cognitive, functional, behavioral, and global outcome measures. New, potentially disease-modifying therapies now in preclinical or clinical studies may be more effective in preventing or arresting the progression of AD and will also test the amyloid hypothesis discussed in this section.[146]

Anti-Inflammatory Drugs

Brain inflammation is a hypothesized cause of neuronal injury in AD. Data have shown that anti-inflammatory drugs may act as protective agents.[26] However, more placebo-controlled trials are needed to test this possibility and to find whether this proposed benefit is a class effect of the nonsteroidal anti-inflammatory drugs or if it is restricted to specific agents.

Statins

In a Cochrane review of studies on statins published in 2001, the reviewers concluded that there is currently no good evidence that statins reduce the risk of Alzheimer's disease.[146] There is, however, a growing body of biological, epidemiological, and some nonrandomized clinical evidence that lowering serum cholesterol may slow the development of Alzheimer's disease.[27]

Clinical studies to determine the potential benefit of statin therapy should be a high priority for future research agendas.

Amyloid-Modifying Agents

The amyloid cascade hypothesis states that Aβ-42 plays an early and crucial role in all cases of AD. A greater understanding of the importance of Aβ in the pathogenesis of AD has led to the investigation of a number of potential anti-amyloid therapies.

Tramiprosate

Tramiprosate is in the most advanced stage of development. It is a glycosaminoglycan (GAG) mimetic designed to interfere with the actions of Aβ early in the cascade of amyloid-producing events.

Preclinical data have shown that tramiprosate reduces brain and plasma levels of Aβ, prevents fibril formation, and shows protective effects in the brain. Phase II clinical trials show improvement or stabilization of cognitive function symptoms, findings confirmed by open-label extensions of these studies. In these trials, tramiprosate appears to be well tolerated with no reports of safety concerns.[147] Phase III trials are ongoing.

Tarenflurbil

Tarenflurbil or R-flurbiprofen is the single enantiomer of the nonsteroidal anti-inflammatory drug flurbiprofen. It modulates rather than inhibits r-secretase activity and results in a reduction of Aβ-42 levels.[148,149]

A randomised Phase II trial showed that tarenflurbil at a dose of 800 mg twice daily was well tolerated by patients with mild AD who showed less decline in activities of daily living and global function.[150]

However, a Phase III clinical trial of tarenflurbil in 1800 patients with mild AD for 18 months showed no statistically significant benefit versus placebo on either cognition or activities of daily living, and therefore further development of the product was stopped by Mydriad Genetics.[151]

Secretase Inhibitors

Blocking the production of Aβ-42 is a major focus of research in AD drug therapy. The identification of beta-secretase, the enzyme that generates a crucial part of Aβ-42, has made it one of the main AD targets. Although inhibition of beta-secretase holds great promise in AD pharmacotherapy, the unusual biology of this enzyme will make the drug-development process challenging.[152]

Immune Therapies

Immunotherapy targeting Aβ has demonstrated a remarkable capacity to arrest and even reverse elements of the brain pathology in AD. Immune therapies include the Alzheimer's disease vaccine and intravenous immunoglobulin (IVIg) infusion.

Several companies are now looking at different versions of active anti-amyloid vaccine and passive immunization approaches involving monoclonal antibodies against Aβ peptides for patients with AD.

Alzheimer's Disease Vaccine

Some vaccines aim to trigger production of antibodies that destroy plaques containing Aβ by injecting the protein into muscles. Earlier clinical trials of such vaccines were stopped because of the development of meningoencephalitis in some patients.[153]

A 2006 publication discussed the safety and efficacy of a new DNA vaccine against Alzheimer's disease. It used a stretch of DNA that codes for the Aβ peptide, instead of using the peptide itself, to stimulate antibody production. The mice that were used were engineered to develop Alzheimer's-like symptoms by producing Aβ peptides in the brain, which in turn form the plaques that lead to cognitive impairment. These APP23 mice were injected with the DNA vaccine before Aβ peptides had started to build up. The DNA vaccine reduced Aβ burden to 15.5% and 38.5%, respectively, of that found in untreated mice at 7 and 18 months of age. In a second part of the study, therapeutic treatment using the vaccine in mice that already had Aβ deposits resulted in reduction of burden to approximately 50% at the age of 18 months. On a promising note, this therapy did not cause neuronal injury or T-cell responses, even after long-term vaccination. The results could signal the first safe preventive and therapeutic vaccine for Alzheimer's disease.[154]

Bapineuzumab

Bapineuzumab is humanized monoclonal antibody against Aβ peptides. Currently bapineuzumab is being investigated in a large, placebo-controlled, 18-month Phase III trial in patients with mild to moderate AD. A prior Phase II trial yielded positive results in a subgroup of patients not carrying the APOE4 allele.[155]

Intravenous Immunoglobulin (IVIg)

Intravenous immunoglobulin (IVIg) is obtained from the pooled plasma of healthy blood donors. This product contains natural anti-amyloid antibodies and exhibits potent central nervous system anti-inflammatory properties. IVIg is FDA-approved for the treatment of immune disorders in children and adults and has been used safely in hundreds of thousands of patients. Recent studies showed that IVIg therapy has several positive effects on patients with AD, including improved cognitive functions and lower level of soluble Aβ in the brain. However, the mechanism of action of IVIg is currently unknown.[156,157] Interim analysis of Phase II trials evaluating the safety, efficacy, and biological mechanisms of action of IVIg in mild to moderate AD revealed that over 9 months, patients randomized to IVIg showed significant improvement on a number of cognitive measures compared with placebo. No evidence of toxicity was found.[158]

An NIH-funded Phase III study has been started to determine whether IVIg treatment slows the rate or prevents the decline of dementia symptoms in people with mild to moderate AD.[159]

Neurogenesis Agents

Neurogenesis (formation of new neurons) persists in the aged human dentate gyrus (DG). The DG is part of the hippocampus and is thought to play a crucial part in memory formation and cognition. However, its role in conditions such as Alzheimer's disease is poorly understood. Studies suggest that the development of AD might involve dysregulation of dentate gyrus neurogenesis. Thus, neurogenesis abnormalities are a promising therapeutic target for AD.[160]

Studies show that 5-HT(1A) receptor antagonists can improve cognitive performance, probably by enhancing acetylcholine and glutamate signals in the hippocampus and in cortical areas of the brain.[161] Selective 5-HT(1A) receptor antagonists such as lecozotan may be useful in the treatment of the cognitive deficits seen in Alzheimer's disease. Currently, trials are ongoing to assess the safety, tolerability, and efficacy of lecozotan SR in patients with mild to moderate AD.

Dimebolin

Dimebolin was approved in 1983 as an antihistamine in Russia. Dimebolin inhibits cholinesterases and the NMDA receptor and reduces mitochondrial swelling induced by Aβ. It has been described as a mitochondrial stabiliser.[162]

A Phase II randomized, double-blind, placebo-controlled trial of Dimebolin in 183 patients with mild to moderate AD performed in Russia demonstrated that the drug was statistically significantly superior to placebo on measures of cognition, global impression, activities of daily living, and behavior and was safe and well tolerated.[163] A large, Phase III multinational, randomized, double-blind, placebo-controlled study is nearing completion.

Methylene Blue

Methylene blue is a deep blue dye used in analytical chemistry and in products such as ink. Its trade name is Rember and it has been shown to interfere with tau aggregation.[164]

A Phase II study was done in which 321 people with mild to moderate AD were randomized to treatment with placebo or 30 mg, 60 mg, or 100 mg methylene blue three times daily. After 50 weeks, pooled data from these patients indicated an 81% reduction in the rate of cognitive decline versus controls. The results were highly statistically significant, and the compound was well-tolerated.[165]

How Does Comorbidity Affect Pharmacotherapy Choices for Alzheimer's Disease?

Comorbid Conditions

Several conditions that are more common in the elderly may affect the choice of treatment for AD.

Cardiovascular Disease (CVD)

Many patients with AD also have comorbid cardiovascular disease or risk factors for CVD. Such risk factors include diabetes and increased homocysteine levels. It is important to treat these comorbid conditions by measures such as optimal control of blood pressure and maintenance of a stable blood sugar level. Not doing so can have detrimental effects on cognition. For example, fluctuations in blood sugar levels can cause confusion, which may worsen AD.

All four cholinesterase inhibitors can cause low heart rate (bradycardia) or heart block in patients with cardiac conduction abnormalities.

Hypertension

Memantine given with the antihypertensive drug *hydrochlorothiazide* (HCTZ) can decrease the bioavailability of HCTZ by as much as 20%, leading to possible poor control of blood pressure.[166]

Kidney or Urinary Tract Impairments

Memantine dosage should be decreased to 10 mg daily in patients with severe renal impairment,[166] and galantamine should not be given to these patients.[167] If patients have a severe urinary tract infection or renal tubular acidosis, memantine should be used with caution, as its clearance is reduced. Reduced clearance may increase the risk of side effects.

Digestive Tract Bleeding

Patients with a history of ulcers or those receiving nonsteroidal anti-inflammatory drugs should be monitored for gastrointestinal bleeding if they take any of the four cholinesterase inhibitors.

Asthma or COPD

The cholinesterase inhibitors can worsen airway constriction in patients with asthma or COPD.

Cost of Caring for Alzheimer's Disease Patients With Comorbid Conditions

A 2002 study analyzed the relationship between comorbid conditions and their cost of care for patients with AD and related dementias (ADRD) in a Medicare managed-care organization. The study was a retrospective analysis of administrative data of 3934 patients with ADRD and 19,300 age- and sex-matched controls.[168]

The study found that ADRD patients had more comorbid conditions than patients without dementia. The 10 most prevalent comorbidities in ADRD were:[168]

- ► Cerebrovascular disease
- ► Chronic complications of diabetes
- ► Chronic pulmonary disease
- ► Congestive heart failure
- ► Diabetes
- ► Malignancy
- ► Myocardial infarction
- ► Peptic ulcer disease
- ► Peripheral vascular disease
- ► Renal disease

Prevalence rates of these conditions were significantly higher in ADRD patients than in controls. Costs of care for patients with ADRD and comorbid conditions were substantially higher, compared to costs for controls with the same conditions and no dementia. The authors of this study concluded that AD increases costs through effects on the management of comorbid illnesses.[168] Better management of AD, therefore, would reduce costs of care associated with diseases that are common in the elderly.

Finally, what is good for the heart is good for the brain. That is, there is growing evidence that good control of risk factors for heart attack and stroke may decrease the risk of AD. Positive practices include lowering cholesterol, controlling blood pressure, quitting smoking, losing weight, and exercising.

How Can Alzheimer's Disease Be Prevented Through Lifestyle Modifications?

Risk factors for heart disease such as hyperlipidemia, obesity, hypertension, diabetes, and smoking may also increase a person's long-term risk for Alzheimer's disease. People having two of these risk factors in their early 40s are 70% more likely to be diagnosed with dementia in later life compared to people with none of these risk factors.[169]

Clinical and epidemiological studies have shown that both Type 2 diabetes and hyperinsulinemia are risk factors for the elderly in developing AD.[170] High blood pressure has also been related to pathological manifestations of AD (senile plaques, neurofibrillary tangles, hippocampal atrophy). Also several observational studies have reported that use of antihypertensives decreases risk of AD.[171]

High-fat diets and sedentary lifestyles have led to a growing incidence of obesity, dyslipidemia and high blood pressure, and these health conditions develop along with, or may be precursors to atherosclerosis, cardiovascular disease, and diabetes. Recent studies have found that most of these disorders can also be linked to an increased risk of AD.[172] Several prospective studies have found associations between intake of dietary fats and risk of AD. High intake of saturated and transunsaturated (hydrogenated) fats was positively associated with increased risk of AD; intake of polyunsaturated and monounsaturated fats protected against cognitive decline in elderly people.[173,174] In a 4-year follow-up of 980 elderly people, risk of AD was higher among those with high fat and calorie intake who had the APOE4 allele.[175]

Dietary modification such as reduced fat intake and reduced salt intake and lifestyle modification to include daily physical and mental activity, may delay the onset and/or decrease the risk of developing AD.

Higher baseline body mass index (BMI) and slower declining BMI in late life are associated with a reduced risk of AD.[175,176] A study done examining the association between midlife BMI and risk of both AD and vascular dementia an average of 36 years later found that compared to those with a normal BMI (18.5–24.9), those obese (BMI ≥ 30) at midlife had a 3.10-fold increase in risk of AD, while those overweight (BMI ≥ 25 and < 30) had a twofold increase in risk of AD and vascular dementia.[177]

Thus, reducing weight during midlife may reduce the risk of developing Alzheimer's disease.

Chapter Summary

The known deficiencies in cholinergic neurons in AD led to the development of cholinesterase inhibitors (ChEIs) for symptomatic treatment of the disease. ChEIs may slow down the decline of patients with AD, but they do not reverse the course of the disease. Memantine (Namenda), an NMDA receptor antagonist, is another medication indicated for the treatment of patients with AD.

The ChEIs that are FDA-approved for treating AD are tacrine (Cognex, rarely used because of hepatotoxicity), rivastigmine (Exelon, also available as a transdermal patch), donepezil

(Aricept), and galantamine (Razadyne, also available in an extended-release formulation as Razadyne ER). The ChEIs are indicated for mild to moderate AD. Donepezil is also indicated for moderate to severe AD, as is the NMDA receptor antagonist memantine.

Investigative medications for AD include selective amyloid-β–lowering agents such as tramiprosate, secretase inhibitors, and intravenous immunoglobulins.

Currently, there is no proven effective treatment for behavioral and psychological symptoms of dementia. ChEIs and memantine seem to improve BPSD symptoms in AD patients. Studies with antipsychotics (first and second generation) and anticonvulsants have yielded no conclusive measurable benefits to date.

Chapter Four
Psychosocial Treatments for Alzheimer's Disease

This chapter answers the following:

▶ **What Psychosocial Interventions Are Used to Treat BPSD in Patients With Alzheimer's Disease, and How Effective Are They?** This section covers psychosocial and environmental interventions for treating BPSD in patients with Alzheimer's disease. Their efficacy is also discussed.

▶ **What Other Therapeutic Interventions Can Be Tried in Patients With Alzheimer's Disease?** This section reviews other therapeutic interventions that have been tried in patients with Alzheimer's disease.

In addressing the BPSD present in more than half of patients with Alzheimer's disease, psychosocial and environmental interventions should be used as the first treatment choice and prior to pharmacological treatments. This is true especially in nonurgent situations.

Risk factors for BPSD can be classified as modifiable or non-modifiable.

Modifiable risk factors for BPSD include:[178]

▶ Lack of caregiver preparedness
▶ Multiple medications
▶ Chaotic living conditions

Nonmodifiable risk factors for BPSD include:

▶ Multiple comorbid conditions
▶ Degree of dementia
▶ Preexisting personality disorder

What Psychosocial Interventions Are Used to Treat BPSD in Patients With Alzheimer's Disease, and How Effective Are They?

There is some evidence that approaches such as games, pet therapy, recreational therapies using crafts, and therapies using dance and art decrease behavioral problems and improve mood.[179–181]

In addition to traditional psychosocial interventions, new methods are emerging for the treatment of different BPSD symptoms. Nontraditional methods such as music therapy, massage, and simulated presence are emerging alongside the more tried-and-true methods of cognitive therapy, occupational therapies, and positive reinforcements. Treatment methods and efficacy are discussed next for each BPSD symptom.

Depression

Nonpharmacological methods to combat depression include cognitive therapy and new methods such as music therapy and therapeutic physical activity. Additionally, behavioral interventions for both patients and caregivers are showing promise in reducing depression in both groups.

Cognitive Therapy: This therapy, used with adults exhibiting mild dementia, challenges the patient's negative ideations. Several randomized, controlled trials using cognitive stimulation therapy have shown reduction in depressive symptoms.[182]

In cognitive therapy, patients identify and record unhelpful thoughts that increase their negative feelings (such as the sense of helplessness). The therapist then helps them find more productive, alternative thoughts. For example, the therapist might help the patient concentrate on what he or she *can* do, instead of on the patient's deficits. The therapist also helps the patient stay grounded in the present. Before and after exploring positive alternatives to negative thoughts, patients are asked to rate their feelings. This process gives them a sense of control and accomplishment.

> **Case Example**
> A patient with AD is no longer able to correctly handle her finances. The patient feels depressed and in her mind magnifies this deficit until she is convinced it is the worst thing that can happen to anybody. She feels hopeless. The therapist then makes the patient challenge her belief and explore adaptive alternatives, such as by saying, *"This is just one thing I can't do. I am still good at doing other things, like cooking."*

Cognitive Stimulation Therapy: This approach attempts to provide a stimulating learning environment in a group situation. A blackboard used during the sessions helps the patients focus and reminds them why they are there. The program stresses information processing over factual knowledge. For example, the patients may be presented with photos of famous faces, but instead of being asked to recognize each face (factual knowledge), the patients are asked questions such as "Who looks youngest?" (information processing).

Behavioral Intervention: This form of therapy, used in patients with moderate or severe dementia, aims to increase the level of the patient's positive activities and interactions and decrease negative ones.[183]

In a study of nonpharmacological treatment of depression in patients with Alzheimer's disease, two behavioral treatments were compared under typical care and control conditions of equal duration. One behavioral treatment emphasized pleasant events for the patient, and the other emphasized caregiver problem-solving. Seventy-two patient–caregiver pairs were randomly assigned to one of the four study arms and were assessed at pretreatment, posttreatment, and 6-month follow-up appointments. Patients in both behavioral treatment programs showed significant improvement in depression symptoms over those in the two control arms. These gains remained at the 6-month follow-up. Caregivers in each behavioral program also showed significant improvement in their own depressive symptoms, while caregivers in the control arms did not. These results show that behavioral interventions for depression are important and effective strategies for treating patients with dementia and their caregivers.[184]

Therapeutic Activity: These programs may also help in treating depression in patients with AD. A study of residents with dementia in a long-term care facility used a wheelchair bicycle in a protocol that combined small group activity therapy and one-on-one bike rides with a staff member.[185] Depression levels in enrolled residents were significantly reduced in the 2-week active portion of the study. This improvement was sustained throughout the 10-week maintenance period. In addition to documenting reduced depression levels, the authors also noted improvements in sleep patterns and in levels of participation in activities.

Music Therapy: This approach also has evidence of support in the treatment of depression in patients with AD. Small studies found that music therapy might help to reduce depressive symptoms in elderly persons with dementia.[186,187] One case study also found that music therapy helped a patient with AD overcome many negative emotions in adjusting to life at a long-term care facility.[188]

Anxiety

There is some evidence that music therapy and group cognitive therapy may reduce anxiety in patients with AD.[189,192] In addition, treating caregivers' depression and anxiety seems to have a positive effect on the patient's anxiety level.

A 2000 study looked at the effects of group intervention for caregivers on the AD patients themselves.[190] Interventions included cognitive behavior therapy, modeling, and knowledge dissemination. The results showed a significant improvement in the anxiety levels of the patients, demonstrating that psychological/educational group interventions for caregivers are helpful for the patients as well.

Staff members in facilities taking care of patients with AD should be aware of their own challenges when caring for these patients. For example, facility caregivers should control the urge to rush AD patients during basic daily activities such as feeding and bathing. These patients need more time to complete these tasks than do other patients, including other adult psychiatric patients. Training staff members in integrity-promoting care can also improve the patient's anxiety.[191] Integrity-promoting care should also include efforts by the nursing staff to make the patient's environment more homelike (for example, by hanging family pictures in the patient's room).

Wandering

There are different types of wandering patterns with different etiologies, which include both emotional and physiological origins. All interventions should focus on understanding why the behavior is present.[193] Wandering may provide several benefits for the patient with AD, such as satisfying emotional needs or improving physical conditions. For example, wandering may improve poor circulation and oxygenation or ease the pain of contractures. Management of the patient's surroundings is the best method of dealing with wandering behavior. This means providing a safe environment where wandering can be tolerated, not medicated.

In a small study, clinicians observed the wandering behavior of four patients with dementia residing in a long-term care facility. They identified the benefits these patients were deriving from wandering (attention, sensory stimulation, or tangible goods such as sweets). These benefits were then given to the patients only during intervals of no wandering as a differential reinforcement of other behavior (DRO). Significant reductions in wandering (> 60% for all patients) were observed. Wandering started again when benefits were applied only during wandering phases and decreased significantly again when DRO was reinstated.[194]

Visually changing the environment and unlocking doors are other methods that may reduce wandering behavior. In a 1995 study, in an attempt to control a problem of patients with dementia exiting a special care unit, the investigators changed the patients' views and light levels from windows using window blinds, cloth barriers concealing the door knobs, or a combination of the two. The cloth barrier proved the most effective solution, reducing exiting due to wandering by 96%. The other methods reduced exiting as well, though to lesser degrees.[195]

One small, uncontrolled study examined the effect on wandering of opening ward doors for 3-hour periods. Patients showed a decreased tendency to wander when the door was open.[196] Another study looking at four patients with AD dementia found that a black horizontal grid on the door reduced the patients' contact with the door by up to 97%.[197]

Case Presentation: Mrs. S. G.

Mrs. S. G. is a 71-year-old patient with advanced AD. She lives at home, and her 76-year-old husband is her primary caregiver. Her deteriorating condition takes a considerable emotional toll on Mr. G. He tells his primary care physician that he has no energy lately, no enthusiasm, and, on top of that, his wife is starting to wander away from home.

"I don't know what to do," he said tearfully. "I'm afraid I might have to put her in a home, and I promised her I wouldn't when she first got sick."

The physician suggests that Mr. G. needs a break. Since the couple's children are unable to care for their mother full-time, she is admitted to a residential facility for 9 days, while Mr. G. visits their favorite vacation spot. He returns with more energy and enthusiasm than he had. Back home with his wife, he shares his vacation stories with her and reminisces about the vacations they took to the same place. He tells his physician that he is paying more attention to his wife now.

"She likes the stories and smiles at the pictures," he reports. Best of all, he adds, her wandering stopped with his renewed attention.

Apathy

A randomized, controlled, partially masked, small study (37 patients) compared a kit-based activity intervention to spending one-on-one time with an activity therapist. The primary outcome measure was the Apathy score of the Neuropsychiatric Inventory (NPI). Both methods resulted in significant improvement in apathy scores on the NPI. There was no clear advantage to one therapy over the other.[198] More research is needed to develop specific behavioral interventions for apathy in patients with dementia.

Agitation

Agitation in patients with dementia commonly falls into three categories[199]

1. *Spontaneous agitation* most frequently occurs in the evenings and has no apparent cause. Increased daytime activities, avoidance of caffeine, and having no naps during the day may decrease the chances of spontaneous agitation.

2. *Reactive agitation* is, as the name implies, agitation in response to an event such as a change in routine or an argument with a caregiver. Caregiver education and a strong support system can help minimize such agitation, which resembles a temper tantrum.

3. *Disinhibited agitation* may mimic a manic state, is unpredictable, and is usually unrelenting. The patient has no regard for other people's needs. A structured environment with set limits is best suited for a patient with this type of agitation.

Treatments for agitation are becoming more innovative, with therapeutic touch and music therapy supplementing traditional behavioral therapy. Attention to the root cause of the agitation is at the heart of all treatments.

A 1999 study found that an individualized behavioral rehabilitation program resulted in significant behavioral improvement, including in agitation scores, in patients with probable or possible AD. The program included identification of retained ADL skills and habit-training in the performance of these skills.[200]

Investigators evaluated a multicomponent program of cognitive behavior therapy, which included behavioral reinforcement, for managing agitation in probable Alzheimer's disease.[201] The study looked at a man with probable AD who was attending a work program three times a week. The patient's tasks were to fold and collate documents. During the workday, the patient was constantly getting out of his seat and displaying agitated speech, such as making statements about going home. The program's components targeted the specific conditions thought to trigger his agitation, as follows.

Staff members provided behavior-specific praise and a small monetary reward for jobs that were done correctly. In addition, the patient was allowed brief breaks for stretching and snacks every 30 minutes. These breaks were not dependent on his work performance, but reduced the discomfort that accompanied long periods of sitting down. Staff members also allowed the patient to vary his tasks, decreasing boredom by alternating folding and collating every 15 minutes. The fourth component was a visual cue of the patient's progress throughout the day, signifying how many jobs were done and how much time was left until break time or the end of the workday.

When the patient made agitated statements, he was reassured by staff and redirected to his task. The patient was always accompanied by a staff member when he did leave the work room. Overall, the study found a significant reduction in agitated behavior during the treatment period.[201]

Small studies reported significant positive results in reducing agitation with the use of therapeutic touch (including massage), individualized music therapy, and behavioral management techniques that were based on the patients' superstitions. Music therapy also facilitated interaction between patients and reduced agitation.[202–204]

Multisensory stimulation studies employed the Snoezelen multisensory stimulation room. The room is an environment where calm music, aromatherapy, and the use of tactile surfaces and special lighting stimulate the patient's senses. The beneficial effects, however, disappear once treatment stops.[205–206]

Simulated presence is an individualized intervention program for patients with moderate to severe cognitive impairment. Tests identify the patient's most meaningful memories, and an audio system then plays these memories for the patient continuously, simulating live phone calls. Because of the patient's short-term memory deficit, this program can be used over long periods. A study of simulated presence in a nursing home showed it had a positive effect on problem behaviors.[207]

Psychosis

The treating clinician should always explore psychosocial, medical, and environmental causes of delusions and hallucinations in patients with AD. A change in medication may resolve some psychotic symptoms that have a physical cause. Past trauma can sometimes resurface as a delusion. Identifying the trauma and addressing it may help treat the delusional state. Correcting visual and hearing impairments and improving lighting conditions can reduce the risk of visual and auditory misinterpretations seen as hallucinations. Modifying the patient's environment can also be effective, if the environment triggers psychosis. For example, reflections in a mirror or window are sometimes interpreted by the patient as people lying in wait for him or her.[208] Some hallucinations, such as talking to a deceased loved one, comfort the person and do not need to be addressed.[209]

In order to minimize confusion and distress that may come with a delusional state, caregivers should introduce themselves with each encounter. New caregivers should allow older persons some time to become acquainted with them prior to starting care activities.

Capgras syndrome—a delusional belief that a closely related person has been replaced by an impostor

Capgras syndrome is a rare disorder in which a person believes that an identical-looking impostor has replaced someone the patient knows (usually a spouse or other close family member). The disorder is common in psychotic conditions such as schizophrenia, but has also been reported in other patients with certain brain lesions and in AD.

Patients placed in facilities should have frequent contact with family members. This contact can be real (for example, by having visits) or simulated (for example, by using videotapes or items from home).[210]

Some patients with AD believe that someone is stealing their possessions. Methods for helping a patient find personal items can help alleviate this problem. Such methods may include getting multiple copies of reading glasses or purses for the patient.

It is always important to assess the patient with AD and psychosis for depression, because delusions may be linked to depressed affect. In this case, treating depression nonpharmacologically with methods such as increasing levels of positive reinforcements may treat the delusions.

Case Presentation: Mr. O. L.

Mr. O. L. is an 85-year-old WWII veteran with advanced dementia. He has recently started to avoid the dining area in the house, saying enemy soldiers are waiting to ambush him there—he had seen their commander. Through careful, sympathetic questioning, his wife and the home health aide were able to conclude that Mr. O. L. was frightened by his own reflection in the china hutch—he was unable to recognize his own face, and his confusion and dementia led to this paranoid hallucination. His wife covered the glass doors of the hutch with cloth curtains and assured him that the enemy forces had been driven away. Mr. O. L. no longer avoids this area of the house, having assured himself it was "secured by the Allies."

Mrs. L. and the aide avoided arguments, denials, and belittling. They worked together to discover the root of Mr. O. L.'s hallucination and were able to preserve his dignity and the harmony in the house, while resolving a difficult behavioral issue.

Sleep Abnormalities

There is some evidence that bright-light therapy in the evening may improve spontaneous agitation and sleep abnormalities in patients with Alzheimer's disease.[211] Music therapy, such as relaxing music played as patients go to sleep, may also improve sleep in AD patients.[212]

Some clinical and empirical pieces of evidence also support the use of behavioral strategies and physical interventions in treating sleep and nighttime behavioral disturbances in dementia patients. These may include sleep hygiene education, daily walking, and increased light exposure.[213]

The results of a randomized, controlled trial of a comprehensive sleep education program (Nighttime Insomnia Treatment and Education for Alzheimer's Disease [NITE-AD]) were published in 2005.[214] The trial looked at sleep improvements in 36 patients with AD. The patients all lived at home and their families cared for them. All participants received written materials describing both age- and dementia-related changes in sleep and standard principles of good sleep hygiene. Seventeen caregivers received the NITE-AD education and training, while 19 control subjects received only general dementia education and caregiver support. The NITE-AD training included:

- ▶ Daily walks (caregivers were instructed on safely accompanying a person who has AD)
- ▶ Use of a light box for 1 hour per day
- ▶ Reduction of light levels when the patient sleeps
- ▶ Constant bed and wake-up times for the patient
- ▶ Napping time limits of 30 minutes, where naps were not allowed after 1 PM

Caregivers also worked to eliminate factors that were known to awaken the patient at night.

The patients in the NITE-AD group had significantly fewer nighttime awakenings and also spent less total time awake at night after the training. The benefit persisted at the 6-month follow-up. Patients in the treatment group also showed greater improvement in depression ratings than did patients in the control group.

What Other Therapeutic Interventions Can Be Tried in Patients With Alzheimer's Disease?

In AD patients, nonpharmacological therapies can be used to improve quality of life. A discussion of several such therapies follows.

Reminiscence Therapy

reminiscence therapy—participation with another person or group of people in a discussion of past activities, events, and experiences

Reminiscence therapy involves the discussion of past activities, events, and experiences with another person or group of people. These discussions usually include the aid of prompts such as photographs, household items, and other familiar items from the past. Discussion may also include music or past sound recordings.[215] In reminiscence groups, participants with dementia are encouraged to talk about past events at least once a week. Life review usually occurs in individual sessions. In these sessions, the person is guided through life experiences in chronological order and is encouraged to evaluate his or her experiences. The sessions may lead to the creation of a storybook of one's life.

A Cochrane review assessed the effects of reminiscence therapy in people with dementia and their caregivers. The review concluded that "although there are a number of promising indications, in view of the limited number and quality of studies, the variation in types of reminiscence work reported and the variation in results between studies, there is a need for more and better designed trials so that more robust conclusions may be drawn."[215]

Validation Therapy

validation therapy—therapeutic technique that begins with the acceptance of the reality and personal truth of the other person's experience

From 1963 to 1980, Naomi Feil developed *validation therapy* to help older people who suffer from cognitive impairments, and this approach is now also used for people with dementia.[216] The therapist works to affirm the patient's perceptions, regardless of whether these perceptions are realistic. This affirmation thus validates the patient, making him or her feel understood and accepted. It is also important for the therapist to avoid confrontation with the patient; the therapist should assume blame for misunderstandings and leave the session, if needed. Validation therapy in the patient with AD requires more time; the therapist should use a slow pace and redirect patients to a different topic if needed.

A Cochrane review of validation therapy in people with dementia or cognitive impairment found that there is insufficient evidence from randomized trials to draw any conclusions regarding the efficacy of this method.[216]

Reality Orientation

Reality orientation (RO) has its origins in efforts to help severely disturbed war veterans. This technique operates through the presentation of orientation information (i.e., to time, place, and person) in order to provide patients with a greater understanding of their surroundings. Therapists may use watches, calendars, or other visual aids to help orient their clients.

A Cochrane review attempted to assess the evidence for the effectiveness of reality orientation as a classroom-based therapy in elderly persons with dementia. The reviewers concluded that there is some evidence that RO may offer benefits in both cognition and behavior domains in patients with dementia. Further research, according to this review, should examine which features of RO are particularly effective. It is unclear at this time how far the benefits of RO extend after the end of treatment. A continued program may be needed to sustain potential benefits.[217]

reality orientation—therapeutic method that operates through the presentation of orientation information (i.e., to time, place, and person) in order to provide a patient with a greater understanding of his or her surroundings

Chapter Summary

Alzheimer's disease may cause many behavioral and psychological abnormalities in the patient. These symptoms affect not only the patient but also his or her caregiver and other family members. Nonpharmacological techniques can improve or alleviate many of these symptoms, bringing relief to the patient and his or her loved ones.

Cognitive therapy and cognitive behavioral therapy, in its various forms, can be used effectively to combat depression, agitation, and anxiety in patients with mild or moderate AD. Cognitive and behavioral therapies that emphasize the patient's strengths and encourage as much independence as possible seem to achieve the best results. Caregiver education benefits the patient as well, showing effects in areas such as anxiety, agitation, and sleep abnormalities. Educating caregivers also seems to delay placement of the patient in a nursing facility.

Novel techniques such as music therapy, therapeutic massage, and simulated presence are finding their way into the nonpharmacological treatment arsenal for use in all stages of AD. Certain therapeutic methods, such as reality orientation, that were developed for a different population are also being used in the treatment of the AD population, though more studies are needed to determine their effectiveness in AD.

Chapter Five
Ethical, Legal, and Caregiver Issues in Alzheimer's Disease

This chapter answers the following:

▶ **What Are the Important End-of-Life Issues in Alzheimer's Disease?** This section covers important issues that caregivers or family members must address when a patient with Alzheimer's disease enters the final stages of the disease.

▶ **What Are the Important Legal Issues Confronting Families of Patients With Alzheimer's Disease?** This section reviews important legal issues for caregivers or family members of patients with Alzheimer's disease.

▶ **What Are the Important Issues for Caregivers of Patients With Alzheimer's Disease?** This section covers important caregiver issues that all physicians should be aware of, and address, when they treat patients with Alzheimer's disease.

▶ **What Are the Various Care Options for AD Patients?** This section covers various care options that can be used for patients with Alzheimer's disease.

EVERY physician treating patients with Alzheimer's disease should be cognizant of the important end-of-life, legal, and caregiving issues that face patients, their families, and their caregivers.

What Are the Important End-of-Life Issues in Alzheimer's Disease?

Caregivers or family members of patients with Alzheimer's disease often face end-of-life issues that include tough questions, such as:

▶ When should certain treatments stop?

▶ Should the patient receive tube-feeding?

▶ Should hospice care be initiated?

When to Stop Treatments

When the patient with Alzheimer's disease progresses to the terminal phases of the disease and no longer has a meaningful quality of life, cholinesterase inhibitors and memantine should be withdrawn, as should any other nonessential medications such as cholesterol-lowering agents and osteoporosis drugs. While it is appropriate to continue any antibiotic therapy in patients with mild to moderate dementia who require treatment with antibiotics, it should be given to patients with severe dementia only if the patients are well hydrated, can communicate effectively, and are able to walk alone or with assistance. Antibiotics, when used, should be given orally to minimize the discomfort of administration.

Patients with AD who have swallowing problems should not receive sedatives and psychotropic medication; these drugs can reduce consciousness and increase the risk of aspiration pneumonia.

Feeding Issues in Patients With Alzheimer's Disease

Patients with advanced dementia frequently develop eating difficulties that result in weight loss. Doctors often recommend enteral feeding tubes for patients in this situation. The patient with severe dementia faces several risks that practitioners believe might be relieved by enteral feeding, including risks of aspiration pneumonia and pressure sores or infections.[218] However, studies determined that there is a continued risk of aspiration after placement of a feeding tube that appears to result from reflux of gastric contents and aspiration of saliva.[219] In addition, there is a belief that enteral feeding can improve function, prolong survival, or provide palliation. However, there are no data to support the latter views. In fact, some data show that there are *no benefits* to using feeding tubes.[220] Furthermore, there are problems with the use of feeding tubes such as diarrhea, clogging of the tubes, and the tendency of patients with dementia to pull tubes out.[221] (Physical restraints may even be necessary to prevent the patients from pulling out the tubes.) Thus, patients with severe dementia should not be tube-fed.[220]

Hospice Care for Patients With Alzheimer's Disease

Advanced AD can place an immense burden on caregivers as they struggle to provide end-of-life care for patients. Hospice palliative care provides a viable solution. Hospice maintains the patient's quality of life and helps the family during the grieving process and the final stages of a loved one's illness.[222]

Hospice care is for patients with a documented 6 months or less to live. Medicare and some private insurance policies provide reimbursement for this care, whereas Medicaid benefits vary by state. Geriatric psychiatrists can be central in referring families to hospice, and they can remain an important part of the care once it is in place.

Hospice patients are cared for by a multidisciplinary team that includes physicians, nurses, social workers, counselors, and hospice-certified nursing assistants. Also included in the hospice team are members of the clergy, therapists, and volunteers. Each team member provides assistance based on his or her own area of expertise. In addition, hospice provides medications, hospital services related to the terminal stage of AD, and additional helpers in the home, if and when needed.

What Are the Important Legal Issues Confronting Families of Patients With Alzheimer's Disease?

As soon as the diagnosis of Alzheimer's disease is made, the physician should urge counseling of the patient and the family in legal issues, including powers of attorney, guardianship, and living wills. Timely planning eases the burden on the family and assists the physician in the patient's care during the later stages of the disorder.[223]

When a patient with AD becomes unable to make, convey, and carry out decisions required for his or her personal and financial welfare, the need for surrogate decision-making often arises.[224]

Advance Directives

Advance directives fall into two categories: instruction-type directives, such as the living will, and proxy directives, such as the durable *power of attorney* for health care.

Instruction-Type Directives: This document spells out the patient's wishes and instructions with regard to the types of life-sustaining measures that should (and should not) be taken on his or her behalf. These measures include resuscitation, intubation, mechanical ventilation, and tube-feedings.

Proxy Directives: Proxy directives are the various forms of power of attorney, by which the patient with AD can give an individual or institution the authority to act on his or her behalf.

There are three types of power of attorney:

▶ *General Power of Attorney*: A general power of attorney actually terminates when the patient becomes incompetent.

▶ *Springing Power of Attorney*: A springing power of attorney becomes effective only at the time the patient (the principal) becomes incompetent.

advance directives—documents that allow currently competent patients with Alzheimer's disease to stipulate the types of medical procedures they desire once they become mentally incompetent; documents also may provide for legal and financial decision-making to be made on behalf

power of attorney—a document designating another person to act on behalf of the designator; a power of attorney can be limited, for example, to healthcare decisions only; there are several types of power of attorney designations; see *also* advance directives

▶ *Durable Power of Attorney:* A durable power of attorney can become effective upon signing and remains in effect once the principal becomes incapacitated or incompetent.

The Durable Power of Attorney for Health Care designates one or more individuals to make medical decisions on behalf of the patient if he or she should become incompetent.

However, this designation can create problems, especially when it comes to determining competency or lack thereof. Some of the issues that this designation can raise are:[225]

▶ Who determines competency?

▶ How capable is that person?

▶ What criteria are used in making this determination?

▶ Who monitors actions of the designated person to ensure that he or she is making the appropriate medical decisions for the patient?

Table 5.1 presents features of each type of power of attorney.

Guardianship

As the cognitive deficits in a patient with AD become more pronounced (and constitute incompetence) and the patient's capacity for self-management decreases, the need for guardianship increases. Guardianship can be established in the absence of any advance directives and can take precedence

Table 5.1   Differentiation of Power of Attorney Types

	General Power of Attorney	Springing Power of Attorney	Durable Power of Attorney	Durable Power of Attorney for Health Care
Effective Date	Upon signing or at a later date	When the principal becomes incompetent or incapacitated	Upon signing or at a later date	When the principal becomes incompetent or incapacitated
Termination Date	When the principal becomes incompetent or incapacitated	At death or upon revocation if the principal is of sound mind	At death or upon revocation if the principal is of sound mind	At death or upon revocation if the principal is of sound mind
Limitations	May be stipulated	—	May be stipulated	For healthcare decisions only

Note: In the context of this publication, the principal is the person with AD.

over certain preestablished surrogate arrangements such as the durable power of attorney.

Persons given authority to act on another person's behalf are known as guardians and/or conservators. The most important and most frequently used guardians and conservators are close family members and friends. They are often the people who have known the patients longest and have their loved ones' best interests in mind when making decisions for them.

Guardianship and conservatorship are granted by a judge. The guardian/conservator has the power and authority to make personal and financial decisions for the mentally incompetent person (called the *ward*).

Guardianship of the Person

Guardianship of the person is established in a court hearing, where the guardian is granted the right to make personal decisions for his or her ward.[226] The guardian or guardians can make decisions regarding their ward's living arrangements and medical treatments.

The court can sometimes grant limited, partial, or temporary guardianships, where the limited guardian makes only those personal decisions that the ward is incapable of making. The limits are specified by the court. The issue of limited guardianship is especially important in view of the waxing and waning nature of mental capacity in many patients with Alzheimer's disease, who may have the ability to rationally make certain kinds of decisions but not others.

Conservatorship

Conservatorship of the estate is also established in a court hearing. It empowers one party (the *conservator*) to control the property of another person and to make financial decisions for that person.[226]

Estate refers to the assets owned by the ward and consists of all items of real property, such as a house or land, and of personal property, such as vehicles and stock. The conservator is responsible for all the assets in the estate.

Sometimes the patient with AD is capable of participating in some financial decisions. In this case, the conservator performs only tasks that are beyond the capacity of the patient with AD and permits the patient to manage other financial tasks that remain within his or her abilities.

What Are the Important Issues for Caregivers of Patients With Alzheimer's Disease?

Stress

Compared with caregivers of people without dementia, caregivers of patients with dementia spend many more hours per week providing care, and the care they provide has a greater impact on their employment, mental and physical health, and family relationships.[227] Studies have shown that family caregivers of relatives with Alzheimer's disease are at a high risk for psychological distress, where their rates of clinical depression and depressive symptoms are far in excess of those in an age-matched population.[228] Caregiver stress can also lead to violence toward the patient.

Data also suggest that although stress and negative affect decrease in caregiving spouses after the deaths of their loved ones with AD, the spouses' scores on depression, loneliness, and positive affect scales do not rebound to levels comparable with an age-matched population. In fact, their scores remain similar to those of current caregivers for up to 3 years after caregiving has ceased. It is clear that some consequences of long-term caregiving may be enduring as well, and it is important that the needs of caregivers be recognized and addressed.[229]

Case Presentation: Ms. G. V.

When my mom, who has Alzheimer's disease, moved in with us, life became almost unbearable overnight. She lived on her own until it was no longer safe for her to do so. When we took her in, she needed a lot of care and watching. My husband and I both work outside the home, and the kids are in high school. It was hard enough for all of us to watch her mind disappear. But the day-to-day logistics made me feel, sometimes, as if I couldn't cope. If I take Mom to an afternoon doctor's appointment, who will take Kathy to her swim meet? My husband had to take Jason to the orthodontist on the same day . . . Who is going to watch Mom during work and school hours to make sure she doesn't accidentally set the house on fire, something she's almost done in her own apartment several times? The questions kept me up at night and my job performance suffered, which of course led to more anxiety—if I lost my job, how would we afford mom's care, Jason's braces, Kathy's guitar lessons . . . I felt like a gerbil on that endless spinning wheel.

Luckily, my mother's doctor helped us find a support group in our area. And the group pointed us to resources we never knew existed. But until then, I really thought I'd end up institutionalized myself!

Role of Caregiver Education in Delaying Institutionalization

It is important to educate caregivers of patients with Alzheimer's disease.

A community study of 406 spouses who were caregivers of patients with AD evaluated the efficacy of a counseling and support program for caregivers. The criterion of efficacy was the length of time until the patient's placement in a nursing home compared against a model prediction.[230] Participants received six sessions of individual and family counseling, took part in a support group, and were able to utilize telephone counseling when needed. Response to the program was evaluated through the use of structured questionnaires, which were administered at baseline, every 4 months for the first year, and every 6 months thereafter. The study enrolled families over a 9.5-year period.

Family members learned to support caregivers and communicate effectively. The caregivers and other family members were also taught to share chores, lessening the burden on the primary caregiver. Caregivers were taught to capitalize on the patient's remaining strengths and to keep the environment safe for the patient.

The primary caregivers (spouses) were taught effective communication methods with the patient, including:

- ▶ Using simple language
- ▶ Maintaining eye contact with the patient
- ▶ Keeping their voices calm

The patients whose spouses received intervention had a lower nursing home placement rate than did patients with spouses in the control group, who received no intervention. In the intervention group, the median difference between predicted and actual time to nursing home placement was 557 days. Caregivers reported improvements in their satisfaction with their support network and felt better able to handle the patients' behavior problems. They also reported improvements in their depression symptoms. These improvements were the biggest factors affecting delay in placement. Thus, it is clear that better practical and emotional support for caregivers could yield considerable benefits for everyone touched by AD, including the patient.

Resources for Caregivers of Patients With Alzheimer's Disease

The following are various resources that may be used by caregivers of patients with Alzheimer's disease.

1. *Support groups* are free and open to caregivers of patients with Alzheimer's disease. They provide caregivers with the understanding, coping mechanisms, and practical tips needed for managing AD. The Alzheimer's Association has information about local support groups in the caregiver's area.

2. *Adult daycare services* provide social and recreational activities, meals, and, if needed, nursing care for patients. The centers will individualize treatment plans and provide transportation to and from their facilities. They may also offer support groups for caregivers.

3. *In-home care agencies* provide services such as personal care, companion services, household assistance, and skilled nursing care.

4. *Independent companions* can provide services such as housekeeping, cooking, and personal care.

5. *Local Alzheimer's disease associations* sometimes have respite care assistance programs that provide eligible caregivers with a small monthly stipend. The stipend helps caregivers hire someone to help them with caregiving duties, allowing them to take time off.

Support Groups

Participation in support groups and counseling may lead to sustained benefits in terms of reducing depressive symptoms in caregivers of patients with Alzheimer's disease.[231] Many support groups are available, including ones supported by the Alzheimer's Association (online at www.alz.org).

What are the Various Care Options for Patients With Alzheimer's Disease?

Adult Daycare Centers

Many people who care for patients with AD also work and are unable to stay home the whole day to care for a loved one. In addition, caregivers like to have some help with care, time to do household work, or just free time for themselves. At such times, adult daycare centers can be used. Patients with AD can attend daycare centers for a few hours a day or the whole day, one or more days per week, if needed. In daycare centers, patients get meals and receive health screenings and monitoring, assistance with activities of daily living, and physical therapy. Most daycare centers provide transportation, an added advantage for the busy caregiver.

Case Presentation: Mr. S. F.

Mr. S. F. is a 78-year-old widower with early AD. He now lives with his son and his son's family. Although he is fairly independent, his forgetfulness and increasing difficulty with decision-making caused several near disasters in the family's home. Since Mr. S. F.'s son and daughter-in-law work outside the home, they desperately needed a solution that would be financially feasible and would satisfy everyone involved. Although services were not covered by Medicaid, the family found the local adult daycare center to be affordable. After initially resisting the idea loudly, Mr. S. F. now says:

The center is different from what I had expected. I've been there a month and I already made some great friends among the staff and other clients. We have fun all day—I'm almost dreading the boredom at Greg's house in the evening. I actually think my memory has gotten a little better since I started going—the first week, I kept forgetting when to be ready for the van. In the last 3 weeks, I remembered to be ready on time most days.

Assisted Living

Some patients with moderate AD need continuous assistance with activities of daily living, as well as assistance with medications. These patients would benefit from assisted living arrangements. Assisted living facilities are appropriate for patients who do not require the continuous skilled nursing care that nursing homes provide.

Patients with AD stay in assisted living facilities instead of at home. They get help with activities such as meals, bathing, grooming, and taking medications. Meals are provided to the residents in a common dining area, and housekeeping and laundry services are available on-site. Other services are also available, such as recreational activities. Security and staff are available around the clock.

Case Presentation: Ms. J. C.

My mother and I always had a strained mother–daughter relationship, so when we were told she had "probable mild Alzheimer's disease," we both felt that living together was not going to work. She is a very proud, independent woman. The diagnosis itself was a harsh blow to all of us, but when she landed in the hospital because she forgot to take the insulin for her diabetes, things got worse. There was a lot of stress involved in trying to find a solution that would let my mom keep her independence, while at the same time ensuring that she was physically safe. Assisted living is a great solution. She's met some people there that she likes to spend time with, the facilities are nice and clean, and keeping her independence really cheered her up. We are now better able to focus on planning for the future and making the most of the good days we have left.

Nursing Homes

At some point, patients with AD may need continuous, 24-hour care. When such care cannot be provided by the usual caregivers, patients can benefit from placement in nursing homes.

Studies have shown that predictors of nursing home placement for patients with dementia are:[232]

> ▶ Increasing severity of dementia

> ▶ Increasing number of comorbid diseases

> ▶ Increasing need for daily assistance

> ▶ Increasing age

Studies have also shown that the reasons given by caregivers for placing patients in nursing homes include:[233]

> ▶ Patients' needs for more skilled care

> ▶ Worsening of caregiver health

> ▶ Patients' dementia-related behaviors

> ▶ Caregivers' needs for more assistance

Behavioral problems are most often cited as the reason for placement.[234]

Nursing homes can be either skilled nursing facilities, providing 24-hour nursing care and medical coverage for patients with AD, or intermediate care facilities. The latter provide health-related care for patients with AD who do not require 24-hour medical and nursing supervision. Nursing care in nursing homes is provided at all times, as needed. If skilled care is required, registered nurses and physical and respiratory therapists are available to provide it, and the care is supervised and authorized by primary care physicians and psychiatrists.

All nursing homes are inspected regularly for quality of care by their state and federal authorities. Inspection reports of all facilities are available online at www.medicare.gov.

Special Care Units

Patients with AD who are in advanced stages or who have more severe cognitive, behavioral, and functional deficits are often placed in special care units.[235]

Special care units are tailored to the specific needs of each patient and have specially trained, professional staff skilled in handling the behaviors typical of these patients. Special care units for patients with AD also have features that utilize environmental cues to decrease BPSD; they may use color-coded hallways, for example, to orient patients to their environment. Patients are also offered freedom to move about in an unrestricted space within the AD special care unit.

Table 5.2 summarizes the features of care arrangements not provided by family or other caregivers.

Table 5.2   Care Options for Patients With AD

Adult daycare centers
- Are for patients in early stages of AD
- Provide respite for caregivers
- Are a viable solution for caregivers who also work outside the home
- Provide a social environment and appropriate care

Assisted living
- Is for patients not requiring constant care
- Provides assistance with meals, grooming, and basic health care
- Allows patients to live independently in a supervised environment
- Is unregulated at the federal level

Nursing homes
- Are for patients requiring constant care that they cannot get at home and/or for those requiring skilled medical care
- Can be either a skilled nursing facility that provides constant medical care or an intermediate care facility where skilled nursing is not constantly required
- Are usually regulated and licensed

Special care units
- May exist within a nursing home or in a hospital
- Are for patients with particularly difficult cognitive or behavioral issues

Hospice care
- May be in-home or residential
- Provides palliative care only
- Is for patients in end-stage AD, with less than 6 months' life cxpcctancy
- Provides a multidisciplinary team to support the patient and family; support includes respite care and spiritual care

Chapter Summary

Alzheimer's disease presents many challenges to patients, their families, and their caregivers (who are often family members). Caregiver stress is a bigger problem among those caring for patients with AD than among those caring for people without AD. Caregiver stress can translate into early placement of the patient in a nursing facility or violence toward the patient. It is therefore important to educate caregivers and other family members about resources available to them (including respite care and day centers), about effective communication with the patient and each other, and about fair sharing of the responsibilities of caregiving.

As the patient's condition worsens, difficult questions face the family. The first is whether to place the patient in assisted-living or nursing facilities. Others involve the end-of-life issues such as when to withdraw treatments and whether to start hospice care. It is important that while patients are still mentally competent, issues such as advanced medical directives, guardianship, and conservatorship be discussed and agreed upon.

Appendix
Resources for Caregivers and Physicians

Resources for Caregivers

Internet Resources

- ▶ Alzheimer's Association—www.alz.org
- ▶ Geriatric Mental Health Foundation—www.gmhfonline. org
- ▶ Alzheimer Research Forum—www.alzforum.org
- ▶ Alzheimer's Disease Education and Referral Center at the National Institute on Aging—http://www.nia.nih. gov/Alzheimers/
- ▶ American Association for Geriatric Psychiatry—www.aagpgpa.org
- ▶ International Psychogeriatric Association—www.ipa-online.org
- ▶ The official Medicare Web site—www.medicare.gov
- ▶ ARCH National Respite Network—www.archrespite. org
- ▶ National Adult Day Services Association—www.nadsa. org
- ▶ Alzheimer's Resource Room of the Department of Health and Human Services Administration on Aging—www.aoa.gov/
- ▶ List of the National Institute on Aging Alzheimer's Disease Research Centers, by state—www.nia.nih.gov/ Alzheimers/ResearchInformation/ResearchCenters
- ▶ The Alzheimer's Disease Clinical Trials Database—www.nia.nih.gov/Alzheimers/ResearchInformation/ ClinicalTrials
- ▶ Family Caregiver Alliance—www.caregiver.org
- ▶ National Family Caregivers Association—www.nfcacares.org

Books and Articles

- ▶ *The 36-Hour Day: A Family Guide to Caring for Persons with Alzheimer Disease, Related Dementing Illnesses, and Memory Loss in Later Life* by Nancy L. Mace, MA, and Peter V. Rabins, MD, MPH
- ▶ "Forget me not: Advances in Alzheimer's disease" by Peg Gray-Vickrey, RNC, DNS, in *Nursing* 2002

▶ *The Memory Bible: An Innovative Strategy for Keeping Your Brain Young* by Gary Small, MD

▶ *Alzheimer's from the Inside Out* by Richard Taylor, PhD

Internet Resources for Physicians

▶ Geriatric Depression Scale (GDS)—www.stanford.edu/~yesavage/GDS.html

▶ Psychological Assessment Resources (publishers of the MMSE)—www3.parinc.com

Glossary

A

acetylcholine—a neurotransmitter that seems to be heavily involved in processes involving learning and memory; its availability is significantly reduced in AD

activities of daily living (ADLs)—daily activities one carries out, from basic activities, such as self-care, to more complex activities, such as paying bills or balancing a checkbook

advance directives—documents that allow currently competent patients with Alzheimer's disease to stipulate the types of medical procedures they desire once they become mentally incompetent; documents also may provide for legal and financial decision-making to be made on behalf of the patient

age-associated memory impairment—subjective complaints of memory impairments in an older person despite formal evaluations showing no deficits

agnosia—the inability to recognize sensory cues (sights, sounds, etc.) despite normal intelligence and normal functioning of sensory organs (eyes, ears, etc.)

allele—a form of a gene; for example, the gene for eye color has an allele for blue eyes and an allele for brown eyes

allosteric modulation—the regulation of an enzyme or protein by binding a molecule at a site other than the protein's active site

amygdala—the brain structure important in emotions and reaction to danger

amyloid—a group of complex proteins that share certain laboratory characteristics and form sheets deposited in various tissues under disease conditions

amyloid angiopathy—amyloid deposits in the brain's blood vessels

aphasia—the inability (or impaired ability) to communicate through spoken, written, or sign language; aphasia can refer to the inability to produce such communication or to comprehend it

apolipoprotein E (APOE)—a serum protein important in cholesterol transport; persons with the APOE4 allele are at a higher risk for developing AD, while those with the APOE2 allele seem more protected against the disease

apraxia—(1) the inability to carry out voluntary movements despite intact muscle control; or (2) the inability to use a familiar object despite being able to recognize the object and its intended function

atrophy—wasting away

atypical antipsychotics—second-generation antipsychotic medications with fewer side effects than first-generation medications

B

Babinski sign—a reflex elicited by rubbing the bottom of the foot. It can identify disease of the spinal cord and brain and is also a primitive reflex in infants. When nonpathological, it is called the plantar reflex, whereas Babinski sign refers to the pathological form.

basal forebrain—a brain structure essential to the production of acetylcholine

C

Capgras syndrome—a delusional belief that a closely related person has been replaced by an impostor

cholinergic—relating to or mimicking the action of acetylcholine

comorbid—a disease or condition occurring at the same time as another disease or condition but unrelated to it

C-reactive protein (CRP) level—a measure of inflammatory processes in the body

D

dementia—loss of cognitive and intellectual powers without changes in consciousness

DSM-IV-TR—*Diagnostic and Statistical Manual of Mental Disorders, Fourth Edition, Text Revision*; the standard text setting out the criteria for diagnosing mental disorders

dysarthria—slurred speech due to muscle weakness, muscle paralysis, or brain injury

E

excitotoxicity—excessive exposure to glutamate or overstimulation of glutamate's membrane receptors

executive functioning—brain functions that allow a person to plan, organize, and carry out goal-oriented behaviors

F

frontal cortex—also known as the prefrontal lobe or cortex, it is the area of the brain largely responsible for executive functions

frontotemporal dementia—dementia affecting the frontal and temporal lobes, causing severe personality changes but few memory deficits

G

glutamate—the most important excitatory neurotransmitter in the brain

H

hippocampus—the brain's memory center; it stores and consolidates memories

homocysteine—an amino acid that is toxic to the body

I

ischemic damage—damage to a part of the body resulting from inadequate blood supply

L

Lewy body dementia (LBD)—dementia distinguished by early psychosis and movement abnormalities as well as characteristic abnormal appearance of neurons in the brain

M

metabolic profile—a series of tests measuring levels of various components of the serum, such as albumin, liver enzymes, and glucose

mild cognitive impairment (MCI)—abnormal short-term memory loss where cognitive functioning remains intact

mixed dementia—concurrent symptoms of two or more types of dementia

N

neuritic plaques—deposits of amyloid in the gray substance of the brain that are associated with destruction of brain structures

neurofibrillary tangles—accumulation of protein fibers twisted within neurons

NMDA receptor—N-methyl-D-aspartate receptor; glutamate receptor

O

omega-3 fatty acids—fatty acids important for maintaining a healthy body and theorized to be protective against AD; omega-3 fatty acids must be obtained through diet, as the body cannot manufacture them

P

parietal cortex—also known as the parietal lobe, this area of the brain receives pain and tactile information; it also analyzes the combined information from the various senses (sight, sounds, taste, etc.)

Parkinson disease dementia (PDD)—dementia in patients with Parkinson disease; occurs in over 50% of patients with Parkinson disease

power of attorney—a document designating another person to act on behalf of the designator; a power of attorney can be limited, for example, to healthcare decisions only; there are several types of power of attorney designations; *see also* advance directives

R

reality orientation—therapeutic method that operates through the presentation of orientation information (e.g., to time, place, and person) in order to provide a patient with a greater understanding of his or her surroundings

reminiscence therapy—participation with another person or group of people in a discussion of past activities, events, and experiences

S

statins—cholesterol-lowering drugs that are hypothesized to protect against AD

sulci—deep grooves on the surface of the brain

T

temporal cortex—also known as the temporal lobe, the part of the brain associated with memories, hearing, and the interpretation of sounds, including spoken language

V

validation therapy—therapeutic technique that begins with the acceptance of the reality and personal truth of the other person's experience

vascular dementia—dementia resulting from infarcts in the brain's blood vessels

ventricle—one of the four chambers in the brain that produce cerebrospinal fluid

References

1. Alzheimer's Foundation of America. About Alzheimer's: Cost. http://www.alzfdn.org/AboutAlzheimers/cost.html. Accessed July 5, 2009.

2. Kamat SM, Taca AC, Grossberg GT. Use of anti-dementia agents: past, present and future. *Primary Psychiatry.* 2004;11(8):56–60.

3. Folstein MF, Folstein SE, McHugh PR. "Mini-mental state." A practical method for grading the cognitive state of patients for the clinician. *J Psychiatr Res.* 1975;12:189–198.

4. Mega MS, Cummings JL, Fiorello T, Gornbein J. The spectrum of behavioral changes in Alzheimer's disease. *Neurology.* 1996;46(1):130–135.

5. Reisberg B, Ferris SH, de Leon MJ, Crook T. The global deterioration scale for assessment of primary degenerative dementia. *Am J Psychiatry.* 1982;139:1136–1139.

6. Reisberg B. Functional assessment staging (FAST). *Psychopharmacol Bull.* 1988;24:653–659.

7. Hebert LE, Scherr PA, Bienias JL, Bennett DA, Evans DA. Alzheimer disease in the U.S. population: Prevalence estimates using the 2000 census. *Arch Neurol.* 2003;60(8):1119–1122.

8. Alzheimer's Association. Alzheimer's Association Report: 2007 Alzheimer's Disease Facts and Figures. http://www.alz.org/national/documents/PR_FFfactsheet.pdf. Accessed July 5, 2009.

9. Desai AK, Grossberg GT. Diagnosis and treatment of Alzheimer's disease. *Neurology.* 2005;64(suppl 3):S34–S39.

10. Grossberg GT, Desai A. Management of Alzheimer's disease. *J Gerontol.* 2003;58A(4):351–353.

11. Evans DA, Funkenstein HH, Albert MS, et al. Prevalence of Alzheimer's disease in community population of older persons: Higher than previously reported. *JAMA.* 1989;262(18):2552–2556.

12. Bird TD, Sumi SM, Nemens EJ, et al. Phenotypic heterogeneity in familial Alzheimer's disease. *Annals of Neurol.* 1989;25(1):12–25.

13. Lautenschlager NT, Cupples LA, Rao VS, et al. Risk of dementia among relatives of Alzheimer's disease patients in the MIRAGE study: What is in store for the oldest old? *Neurology.* 1996;46:641–650.

14. O'Brien JT, Erkinjuntti T, Reisberg B, et al. Vascular cognitive impairment. *Lancet Neurol.* 2003;2:89–98.

15. Schoenberg BS. Epidemiology of dementia. *Neurol Clin.* 1986;4(2):447–457.

16. Levy-Lahad E, Tsuang D, Bird TD. Recent advances in the genetics of Alzheimer's disease. *J Geriatr Psychiatry Neurol.* 1998;11(2):42–54. Review.

17. Corder EH, Saunders AM, Strittmatter WJ, et al. Gene dose of apolipoprotein E type 4 allele and the risk of Alzheimer's disease in late onset families. *Science.* 1993; 261(5123):921–923.

18. Rogaeva E, Meng Y, Lee JH, et al. The neuronal sortilin-related receptor SORL1 is genetically associated with Alzheimer disease. *Nature Genet.* 2007;39(2):168–177.

19. Karlinsky H. Alzheimer's disease in Down's syndrome. A review. *J Am Geriatr Soc.* 1986; 34(10):728–734. Review.

20. Guo Z, Cupples LA, Kurz A, et al. Head injury and the risk of AD in the MIRAGE study. *Neurology.* 2000;54(6):1316–1323.

21. Rondeau V, Commenges D, Jacqmin-Gadda H, Dartiques JF. Relation between aluminum concentrations in drinking water and Alzheimer's disease: An 8–year follow-up study. *Am J Epidemiol.* 2000;152(1):59–66.

22. Green RC, Cupples LA, Kurz A, et al. Depression as a risk factor for Alzheimer disease: The MIRAGE study. *Arch Neurol.* 2003;60: 753–759.

23. Mortimer JA, Snowdon DA, Markesbery WR. Head circumference, education and risk of dementia: Findings from the Nun study. *J Clin Exp Neuropsychol.* 2002; 25(5):671–679.

24. Ravaglia G, Forti P, Maioli F, et al. Homocysteine and folate as risk factors for dementia and Alzheimer disease. *Am J Clin Nutr.* 2005;82(3):636–643.

25. Higgins GA, Large CH, Rupniak HT, Barnes JC. Apolipoprotein E and Alzheimer's disease: A review of recent studies. *Pharmacol Biochem Behav.* 1997;56(4):675–685. Review.

26. McGeer PL, Schulzer M, Mcgeer EG. Arthritis and anti-inflammatory agents as possible protective factors for Alzheimer's disease: A review of 17 epidemiologic studies. *Neurology.*1996; 47(2):425–432.

27. Scott HD, Laake K. Statins for the prevention of Alzheimer's disease. *Cochrane Database Syst Rev.* 2001;(4):CD003160.

28. Pinder RM, Sandler M. Alcohol, wine and mental health: Focus on dementia and stroke. *J Psychopharmacol.* 2004;18(4):449–456. Review.

29. Luchsinger JA, Tang MX, Siddiqui M, Shea S, Mayeux R. Alcohol intake and risk of dementia. *J Am Geriatr Soc.* 2004; 52(4):540–546.

30. Stern Y, Gurland B, Tatemichi TK, Tang MX, Wilder D, Mayeux R. Influence of education and occupation on the incidence of Alzheimer's disease. *JAMA.* 1994;271(13):1004–1010.

31. Wilson RS, Mendes De Leon CF, Barnes LL, et al. Participation in cognitively stimulating activities and risk of incident Alzheimer disease. *JAMA.* 2002;287(6):742–748.

32. Laurin D, Verreault R, Lindsay J, MacPherson K, Rockwood K. Physical activity and risk of cognitive impairment and dementia in elderly persons. *Arch Neurol.* 2001;58(3):498–504.

33. Colcombe SJ, Erickson KI, Raz N, et al. Aerobic fitness reduces brain tissue loss in aging humans. *J Gerontol A Biol Sci Med Sci.* 2003;58:176–180.

34. Verghese J, Lipton RB, Katz MJ, et al. Leisure activities and the risk of dementia in the elderly. *N Engl J Med.* 2003;348:2508–2516.

35. Burns JM, Cronk BB, Anderson HS, et al. Cardiorespiratory fitness and brain atrophy in early Alzheimer disease. *Neurology.* 2008;71(3):210–216.

36. Rolland Y, Pillard F, Klapouszczak A, et al. Exercise program for nursing home residents with Alzheimer's disease: A 1–year randomized, controlled trial. *J Am Geriatr Soc.* 2007;55(2):158–165.

37. Scarmeas N, Stern Y, Tang MX, Mayeux R, Luchsinger JA. Mediterranean diet and risk for Alzheimer's disease. *Ann Neurol.* 2006;59(6):912–921.

38. Morris MC, Evans DA, Bienias JL, et al. Consumption of fish and n-3 fatty acids and risk of incident Alzheimer disease. *Arch Neurol.* 2003;60(7):940–946.

39. McKhann G, Drachman D, Folstein M, Katzman R, Price D, Stadlan EM. Clinical diagnosis of Alzheimer's disease: Report of the NINCDS-ADRDA Work Group under the auspices of Department of Health and Human Services Task Force on Alzheimer's Disease. *Neurology.* 1984;34:939–944.

40. Jost BC, Grossberg GT. The evolution of psychiatric symptoms in Alzheimer's disease: A natural history study. *J Am Geriatr Soc.* 1996;44(9):1078–1081.

41. Olin JT, Schneider LS, Katz IR, et al. National Institute of Mental Health provisional diagnostic criteria for depression of Alzheimer's disease. *Am J Geriatr Psychiatry.* 2002;10:125–128.

42. Jeste DV, Finkel SI. Psychosis of Alzheimer's disease and related dementias: Diagnostic criteria for a distinct syndrome. *Am J Geriatr Psychiatry.* 2000;8(1):29–34.

43. Aarsland D, Cummings JL, Yenner G, Miller B. Relationship of aggressive behavior to other neuropsychiatric symptoms in patients with Alzheimer's disease. *Am J Psychiatry.* 1996;153(2):243–247.

44. Cohen-Mansfield J. Conceptualization of agitation results based on the Cohen-Mansfield Agitation Inventory and the Agitation Behavior Mapping Instrument. *Int Psychogeriatr.* 1996;8(suppl 3):309–315.

45. McCurry SM, Logsdon RG, Teri L, et al. Characteristics of sleep disturbance in community-dwelling Alzheimer's disease patients. *J Geriatr Psychiatry Neurol.* 1999;12(2):53–59.

46. Teri L, Ferretti LE, Gibbons LE, et al. Anxiety of Alzheimer's disease: Prevalence, and comorbidity. *J Gerontol A Biol Sci Med Sci.* 1999;54(7):M348–M352.

47. Chemerinski E, Petracca G, Manes F, Leiguarda R, Starkstein SE. Prevalence and correlates of anxiety in Alzheimer's disease. *Depress Anxiety.* 1998;7(4):166–170.

48. American Psychiatric Association. *Diagnostic and Statistical Manual of Mental Disorders, Fourth Edition, Text Revision.* Washington, DC: American Psychiatric Association; 2000.

49. Sano M. A guide to diagnosis of Alzheimer's disease. *CNS Spectr.* 2004;9(7)(suppl 5):16–19.

50. Tariq SH, Tumosa N, Chibnall JT, Perry MH III, Morley JE. Comparison of the Saint Louis University mental status examination and the mini-mental state examination for detecting dementia and mild neurocognitive disorder—a pilot study. *Am J Geriatr Psychiatry.* 2006;14(11):900–910.

51. Tariq SH, Tumosa N, Chibnall JT, Perry MH III, Morley JE. SLUMS Examination. Department of Veterans Affairs. http://medschool.slu.edu/agingsuccessfully/pdfsurveys/slumsexam_05.pdf. Accessed July 5, 2009.

52. Yesavage JA, Brink TL, Rose TL, et al. Development and validation of a geriatric depression screening scale: A preliminary report. *J Psychiatr Res.* 1983;17:37–49.

53. Mahoney FI, Barthel DW. Functional evaluation: The Barthel Index. *Maryland State Med J.* 1965;2:61–65.

54. Cefalu C, Grossberg G. *Diagnosis and Management of Dementia. American Family Physician Monograph.* No. 2. Leawood, KA: American Academy of Family Physicians; 2001.

55. Seshadri S, Beiser A, Selhub J, et al. Plasma homocysteine as a risk factor for dementia and Alzheimer's disease. *New Engl J Med.* 2002;346:476–483.

56. Duong T, Nikolaeva M, Acton PJ. C-reactive protein-like immuno-reactivity in the neurofibrillatory tangles of Alzheimer's disease. *Brain Res.*1997;749(1):152–156.

57. Engelhart MJ, Geerlings MI, Meijer J, et al. Inflammatory proteins in plasma and the risk of dementia: The Rotterdam study. *Arch Neurol.* 2004;61(5):668–672.

58. Charletta D, Gorelick PB, Dollear TJ, et al. CT and MRI findings among African-Americans with Alzheimer's disease, vascular dementia, and stroke without dementia. *Neurology.* 1995;45(8): 1456–1461.

59. Silverman DH, Small GW, Chang CY, et al. Positron emission tomography in evaluation of dementia: Regional brain metabolism and long-term outcome. *JAMA.* 2001;286:2120–2127.

60. Klunk WE, Engler H, Nordberg A, et al. Imaging brain amyloid in Alzheimer's disease with Pittsburgh Compound-B. *Ann Neurol.* 2004;55(3):303–305.

61. American College of Medical Genetics/American Society of Human Genetics Working Group on ApoE and Alzheimer's Disease. Statement on use of apolipoprotein E testing for Alzheimer's disease. *JAMA.* 1995;274:1627–1629.

62. National Institute on Aging/Alzheimer's Association Working Group. Apolipoprotein E genotyping in Alzheimer's disease. *Lancet.* 1996;347:1091–1095.

63. Borson S, Brush M, Gil E, et al. The clock drawing test: Utility for dementia detection in multiethnic elders. *J Gerontol Med Sci.* 1999;54(11):M534–M540.

64. Lezak MD. *Neuropsychological Assessment.* 3rd ed. New York, NY: Oxford University Press; 1995:1–2.

65. Kertesz A, Clydesdale S. Neuropsychological deficits in vascular dementia versus Alzheimer's disease: Frontal lobe deficits prominent in vascular dementia. *Arch Neurol.* 1994;51:1226–1231.

66. Schmand B, Lindeboom J, Launer L, et al. What is a significant score change on the Mini-Mental State Examination? *Int J Geriatr Psychiatry.* 1995;10:411–414.

67. Jorm AF, Christensen H, Korten AE. Do cognitive complaints either predict future cognitive decline or reflect past cognitive decline? A longitudinal study of an elderly community sample. *Psychol Med.* 1997;27:91–98.

68. Geerling M, Jonker C, Bouter L, et al. Association between memory complaints and incident Alzheimer's disease in elderly people with normal baseline cognition. *Am J Psychiatry.* 1999;156:531–537.

69. Crook T, Bartus RT, Ferris SH, et al. Age-associated memory impairment: Proposed diagnostic criteria and measures of clinical change—report of a NIMH Work Group. *Dev Neuropsychol.* 1986;2:261–276.

70. Gwyther LP. *Care of Alzheimer's Patients: A Manual for Nursing Home Staff.* Chicago: Alzheimer's Association and American Health Care Association; 1985:20–25.

71. Petersen RC, Smith GE, Waring SC, et al. Aging, memory, and mild cognitive impairment. *Int Psychogeriatr.* 1997;9(suppl 1):65–69.

72. Petersen RC, Doody R, Kurz A, et al. Current concepts in mild cognitive impairment. *Arch Neurol.* 2001;58(12):1985–1992. Review.

73. Shah Y, Tangalos EG, Petersen RC. Mild cognitive impairment. When is it a precursor to Alzheimer's disease? *Geriatrics.* 2000;55(9):62, 65–68. Review.

74. Roman GC, Tatemichi TK, Erkinjuntti T, et al. Vascular dementia: Diagnostic criteria for research studies. Report of the NINDS-AIREN International Workshop. *Neurology.* 1993;43:250–260.

75. Cummings JL. Vascular subcortical dementias: Clinical aspects. *Dementia.* 1994;5(3–4):177–180.

76. Sultzer DL, Levin HS, Mahler ME, et al. A comparison of psychiatric symptoms in vascular dementia and Alzheimer's disease. *Am J Psychiatry.* 1993;150(12):1806–1812.

77. McKeith IG, Galasko D, Kosaka K, Perry RH. Consensus guidelines for the clinical and pathologic diagnosis of dementia with Lewy bodies (DLB): Report of the consortium on DLB international workshop. *Neurology.* 1996;47:1113–1124.

78. Barber R, Panikkar A, McKeith IG. Dementia with Lewy bodies: Diagnosis and management. *Int J Geriatr Psychiatry.* 2001;16(suppl 1):S12–S18. Review.

79. Cahn-Weiner DA. Cognitive and behavioral features discriminate between Alzheimer's and Parkinson's disease. *Neuropsychiatry Neuropsychol Behav Neurol.* 2002;15(2):79–87.

80. Aarsland D, Cummings JL, Larsen JP. Neuropsychiatric differences between Parkinson's disease with dementia and Alzheimer's disease. *Int J Geriatr Psychiatry.* 2001;16:184–191.

81. Clinical and neuropathological criteria for frontotemporal dementia. The Lund and Manchester Groups. *J Neurol Neurosurg Psychiatry.* 1994;57:416–418.

82. Reisberg B, Saeed MU. *Alzheimer's Disease. Textbook of Geriatric Psychiatry.* 3rd ed. New York: W.W. Norton and Company; 2004:449–50.

83. Coyle JT, Price DL, DeLong MR. Alzheimer's disease: A disorder of cortical cholinergic innervation. *Science.* 1983;219(4589):1184–1190.

84. Wilkinson DG, Francis PT, Schwam E, Payne-Parrish J. Cholinesterase inhibitors used in the treatment of Alzheimer's disease: The relationship between pharmacological effects and clinical efficacy. *Drugs Aging.* 2004;21(7):453–478. Review.

85. Lipton SA. The molecular basis of memantine action in Alzheimer's disease and other neurologic disorders: Low affinity, uncompetitive antagonism. *Curr Alzheimer Res.* 2005;2(2):155–165.

86. Arai H, Kobayashi K, Ikeda K, et al. A computed tomography study of Alzheimer's disease. *J Neurol.* 1983;229(2):69–77.

87. Wahlund LO. Magnetic resonance imaging and computed tomography in Alzheimer's disease. *Acta Neurol Scand.* 1996;168(suppl):50–53.

88. Aricept [package insert]. New York, NY: Pfizer Inc; 2006.

89. Exelon [package insert]. East Hanover, NJ: Novartis Pharmaceuticals Corp; 2007.

90. Exelon patch [package insert]. East Hanover, NJ: Novartis Pharmaceuticals Corp; 2009.

91. U.S. National Institutes of Health. Comparative efficacy, safety, and tolerability of rivastigmine 10 and 15 cm² patch in patients with Alzheimer's disease (AD) showing cognitive decline. ClinicalTrials.gov Web site. http://www.clinicaltrials.gov/ct/show/NCT00506415. Accessed July 5, 2009.

92. Razadyne [package insert]. Titusville, NJ: Janssen Pharmaceutical Products, LP; 2005.

93. Namenda [package insert]. St. Louis, Mo: Forest Laboratories, Inc; 2003.

94. Grossberg GT, Manes F, Allegri R, et al. A multinational, randomized, double-blind, placebo-controlled, parallel-group trial of memantine extended-release capsule (28 mg, once daily) in patients with moderate to severe Alzheimer's disease. 11th Int Conf Alzheimer's Dis; 2008; Chicago.

95. O'Brien JT, Ballard CG. Drugs for Alzheimer's disease. *BMJ.* 2001;323:123–124.

96. Knapp MJ, Knopman DS, Solomon PR, et al. A 30–week randomized controlled trial of high-dose tacrine in patients with Alzheimer's disease. The Tacrine Study Group. *JAMA.* 1994;271(13):985–991.

97. Birks J, Harvey RJ. Donepezil for dementia due to Alzheimer's disease. *Cochrane Database of Syst Rev.* 2006;1:CD001190.

98. Winblad B, Kilander L, Eriksson S, et al. Donepezil in patients with severe Alzheimer's disease: Double-blind, parallel-group, placebo-controlled study. *Lancet* 2006;367:1057–1065.

99. Birks J, Grimley Evans J, Iakovidou V, Tsolaki M. Rivastigmine for Alzheimer's disease (Cochrane Review). *Cochrane Database Syst Rev.* 2000;(4):CD001191.

100. Farlow MR, Hake A, Messina J, et al. Response of patients with Alzheimer's disease to rivastigmine treatment is predicted by the rate of disease progression. *Arch Neurol.* 2001;58:417–422.

101. Auriacombe S, Pere JJ, Loria-Kanza Y, Vellas B. Efficacy and safety of rivastigmine in patients with Alzheimer's disease who failed to benefit from treatment with donepezil. *Curr Med Res Opin.* 2002;18(3):129–138.

102. Winblad B, Cummings J, et al. IDEAL: a 24 week placebo controlled study of the first transdermal patch in Alzheimer's disease—rivastigmine patch versus capsule. Oral Presentation at the 10th International Congress of Alzheimer's and Related Disorders (ICAD); July 19, 2006; Madrid, Spain.

103. Rockwood K, Mintzer J, Truyen L, et al. Effects of a flexible galantamine dose in Alzheimer disease: A randomised, controlled trial. *J Neurol Neurosurg Psychiatry.* 2001;71(5):589–595.

104. Tariot PN, Solomon PR, Morris JC, et al. A 5–month, randomized, placebo-controlled trial of galantamine in AD. The Galantamine USA-10 Study Group. *Neurology*. 2000;54(12):2269–2276.

105. Loy C, Schneider L. Galantamine for Alzheimer's disease and mild cognitive impairment. *Cochrane Database Syst Rev.* 2006;1:CD001747.

106. Reisberg B, Doody R, Stoffler A, et al; Memantine Study Group. Memantine in moderate-to-severe Alzheimer's disease. *N Engl J Med*. 2003;348(14):1333–1341.

107. Tariot PN, Farlow MR, Grossberg GT, Graham SM, McDonald S, Gergel I; Memantine Study Group. Memantine treatment in patients with moderate to severe Alzheimer disease already receiving donepezil: A randomized controlled trial. *JAMA*. 2004;291(3):317–324.

108. Watkins PB, Zimmerman HJ, Knapp MJ, et al. Hepatotoxic effects of tacrine administration in patients with Alzheimer's disease. *JAMA*. 1994;271:992–998.

109. Grossberg GT, Stahelin HB, Messina JC, et al. Lack of adverse pharmacodynamic drug interactions with rivastigmine and twenty-two classes of medications. *Int J Geriatr Psychiatr.* 2000;15:242–247.

110. Schneider LS, Tariot PN, Dagerman KS, et al. Effectiveness of atypical antipsychotic drugs in patients with Alzheimer's disease. *N Engl J Med*. 2006;355(15):1525–1538.

111. U.S. Food and Drug Administration. Deaths with antipsychotics in elderly patients with behavioral disturbances. http://www.fda.gov/Drugs/DrugSafety/PublicHealthAdvisories/ucm053171.htm. Updated May 7, 2009. Accessed July 5, 2009.

112. De Deyn PP, Katz IR, Brodaty H, et al. Management of agitation, aggression, and psychosis associated with dementia: A pooled analysis including three randomized, placebo-controlled double-blind trials in nursing home residents treated with risperidone. *Clin Neurol Neurosurg.* 2005;107(6):497–508.

113. Street JS, Clark WS, Gannon KS, et al. Olanzapine treatment of psychotic and behavioral symptoms in patients with Alzheimer disease in nursing care facilities: A double-blind, randomized, placebo-controlled trial. The HGEU Study Group. *Arch Gen Psychiatry.* 2000;57(10):968–976.

114. Zhong K, Tariot P, Minkwitz MC, et al. Quetiapine for the treatment of agitation in patients with dementia. [poster]. Presented at: the 158th Annual Meeting of the American Psychiatric Association; May 21–26, 2005; Atlanta, Georgia.

115. De Deyn P, Jeste DV, Swanink R, et al: Aripiprazole for the treatment of psychosis in patients with Alzheimer's disease: A randomized, placebo-controlled study. *J Clin Psychopharmacol*. 2005;25(5):463–467.

116. Dolder CR, Jeste DV. Incidence of tardive dyskinesia with typical versus atypical antipsychotics in very high risk patients. *Biol Psychiatry.* 2003;53(12):1142–1145.

117. Jeste DV, Rockwell E, Harris MJ, et al. Conventional vs. newer antipsychotics in elderly patients. *Am J Geriatr Psychiatry.* 1999;7(1):70–76. Review.

118. Sink KM, Holden KF, Yaffe K. Pharmacological treatment of neuropsychiatric symptoms of dementia: a review of the evidence. *JAMA*. 2005;293(5):596–608.

119. Treatment of agitation in older persons with dementia. Expert Consensus Panel for agitation in dementia. *Postgrad Med.* 1998;Spec No:1–88.

120. Porsteinsson AP, Tariot PN, Erb R, et al. Placebo-controlled study of divalproex sodium for agitation in dementia. *Am J Geriatr Psychiatry.* 2001;9(1):58–66.

121. Tariot PN, Raman R, Jakimovich L, et al. Divalproex sodium in nursing home residents with possible or probable Alzheimer Disease complicated by agitation: A randomized, controlled trial. *Am J Geriatr Psychiatry.* 2005;13(11):942–949.

122. Loy R, Tariot PN. Neuroprotective properties of valproate: Potential benefit for AD and tauopathies. *J Mol Neurosc.* 2002;19(3):303–307.

123. Kim AJ, Shi Y, Austin RC, Werstuck GH. Valproate protects cells from ER stress-induced lipid accumulation and apoptosis by inhibiting glycogen synthase kinase-3. *J Cell Sci.* 2005;118(Pt 1):89–99.

124. U.S. National Institutes of Health. Valproate in Dementia (VALID). ClinicalTrials.gov Web site. www.clinicaltrials.gov/ct/show/ NCT00071721. Accessed July 5, 2009.

125. Tariot PN, Erb R, Leibovici A, et al. Efficacy and tolerability of carbamazepine for agitation and aggression in dementia. *Am J Psychiatry.* 1998;155(1):54–61.

126. Olin JT, Fox LS, Pawluczyk S, Taggart NA, Schneider LS. A pilot randomized trial of carbamazepine for behavioral symptoms in treatment-resistant outpatients with Alzheimer disease. *Am J Geriatr Psychiatry.* 2001;9(4):400–405.

127. Gauthier S, Feldman H, Hecker J, et al. Efficacy of donepezil on behavioral symptoms in patients with moderate to severe Alzheimer's disease. *Int Psychogeriatr.* 2002;14(4):389–404.

128. Figiel G, Sadowsky C. A systematic review of the effectiveness of rivastigmine for the treatment of behavioral disturbances in dementia and other neurological disorders. *Curr Med Res Opin.* 2008;24(1):157–166. Review.

129. Cummings JL, Schneider L, Tariot PN, et al. Reduction of behavioral disturbances and caregiver distress by galantamine in patients with Alzheimer's disease. *Am J Psychiatry.* 2004;161(3):532–538.

130. Cummings JL, Schneider L, Tariot PN, et al. Behavioral effects of memantine in Alzheimer disease patients receiving donepezil treatment. *Neurology.* 2006;67(1):57–63.

131. Grossberg GT, Pejovi V, Miller ML, Graham SM. Memantine therapy of behavioral symptoms in community-dwelling patients with moderate to severe Alzheimer's disease. *Dement Geriatr Cogn Disord.* 2009;27(2):164–172. Epub 2009 Feb 5.

132. Wilcock GK, Ballard CG, Cooper JA, Loft H. Memantine for agitation/aggression and psychosis in moderately severe to severe Alzheimer's disease: A pooled analysis of 3 studies. *J Clin Psychiatry.* 2008;69(3):341–348.

133. Mulnard RA, Cotman CW, Kawas C, et al. Estrogen replacement therapy for treatment of mild to moderate Alzheimer's disease. *JAMA.* 2000;283:1007–1015.

134. Henderson VW, Paganini-Hill A, Miller BL, et al. Estrogen for Alzheimer's disease in women: Randomized, double-blind, placebo-controlled trial. *Neurology.* 2000;54:295–301.

135. Freund-Levi Y, Eriksdotter-Jonhagen M, Cederholm T, et al. Omega-3 fatty acid treatment in 174 patients with mild to moderate Alzheimer disease: OmegAD Study: A randomized double-blind trial. *Arch Neurol.* 2006;63:1402–1408.

136. U.S. National Institutes of Health. DHA (docosahexaenoic acid), an omega 3 fatty acid, in slowing the progression of Alzheimer's disease. ClinicalTrials.gov Web site. www.clinicaltrials.gov/ct2/show/NCT00440050. Accessed July 5, 2009.

137. Alzheimer's Disease Cooperative Study 18–month DHA Trial in Alzheimer's Disease. ICAD 2009: Alzheimer's Association International Conference on Alzheimer's Disease. July 11–16, 2009; Vienna, Austria.

138. Kontush K, Schekatolina S. Vitamin E in neurodegenerative disorders: Alzheimer's disease. *Ann N Y Acad Sci.* 2004;1031:249–262.

139. Sano M, Ernesto C, Thomas RG, et al. A controlled trial of selegiline, alpha-tocopherol, or both as treatment for Alzheimer's Disease Cooperative Study. *N Engl J Med.* 1997;336(17):1216–1222.

140. Kontush A, Mann U, Arlt S, et al. Influence of vitamin E and C supplementation on lipoprotein oxidation in patients with Alzheimer's disease. *Free Radic Biol Med.* 2001;31(3):345–354.

141. Miller ER III, Pastor-Barriuso R, Dalal D, et al. Meta-analysis: High-dosage vitamin E supplementation may increase all-cause mortality. *Ann Intern Med.* 2005;142(1):37–46. Epub 2004 Nov 10.

142. Scarmeas N, Fuchsine JA, Mayeux R, Stern Y. Mediterranean diet and Alzheimer's disease mortality. *Neurology.* 2007;69(11):1084–1093.

143. Sofi F, Cesari F, Abbate R, et al. Adherence to Mediterranean diet and health status: Meta-analysis. *BMJ.* 2008;337:a1344.

144. Scarmeas N, Stern Y, Mayeux R, et al. Mediterranean diet and mild cognitive impairment. *Arch Neurol.* 2009;66(2):216–225.

145. Turner RS. Alzheimer's disease. *Semin Neurol.* 2006;26(5):499–506.

146. Scott HD, Laake K. Statins for the prevention of Alzheimer's disease. *Cochrane Database Syst Rev.* 2001;4:CD003160.

147. Wright TM. Tramiprosate. *Drugs Today (Barc).* 2006;42(5):291–298. Review.

148. Weggen S, Eriksen JL, Sagi SA, et al. Evidence that nonsteroidal anti-inflammatory drugs decrease amyloid beta 42 production by direct modulation of gamma-secretase activity. *J Biol Chem.* 2003;278(34):31831–31837.

149. Weggen S, Eriksen JL, Das P, et al. A subset of NSAIDs lower amyloidogenic Abeta42 independently of cyclooxygenase activity. *Nature.* 2001;414(6860):212–216.

150. Wilcock GK, Black SE, Hendrix SB, et al. Efficacy and safety of tarenflurbil in mild to moderate Alzheimer's disease: A randomised phase II trial. *Lancet Neurol.* 2008;7(6):483–493. Epub 2008 Apr 29.

151. Green RC. Final Phase 3 Results with Tarenflurbil Confirm No Effect in Early AD. ICAD 2008: Alzheimer's Association International Conference on Alzheimer's Disease: Abstract O3–04–01. Presented July 29, 2008. site.

152. Citron M. Beta-secretase inhibition for the treatment of Alzheimer's disease—promise and challenge. *Trends Pharmacol Sci.* 2004;25(2):92–97. Review.

153. Robinson SR, Bishop GM, Munch G. Alzheimer vaccine: Amyloid-beta on trial. *Bioessays.* 2003;25(3):283–288.

154. Okura Y, Miyakoshi A, Kohyama K, et al. Nonviral Abeta DNA vaccine therapy against Alzheimer's disease: Long-term effects and safety. *Proc Natl Acad Scj USA.* 2006;103(25):9619–9624. Epub 2006 Jun.

155. Rafii MS, Aisen PS. Recent developments in Alzheimer's disease therapeutics. *BMC Med.* 2009;7:7. Review.

156. Weksler ME, Gouras G, Relkin NR, Szabo P. The immune system, amyloid-beta peptide, and Alzheimer's disease. *Immunol Rev.* 2005;205:244–256. Review.

157. Istrin G, Bosis E, Solomon B. Intravenous immunoglobulin enhances the clearance of fibrillar amyloid-beta peptide. *J Neurosci Res.* 2006;84(2):434–443.

158. IV Immunoglobulin therapy shows early signs of efficacy in Alzheimer's. ICAD 2008: Alzheimer's Association International Conference on Alzheimer's Disease. July 26–31, 2008; Chicago.

159. U.S. National Institutes of Health. A Phase 3 Study Evaluating Safety and Effectiveness of Immune Globulin Intravenous (IGIV 10%) for the Treatment of Mild to Moderate Alzheimer's Disease. ClinicalTrials.gov Web site. www.clinicaltrials.gov/ct/show/NCT00818662. Accessed July 5, 2009.

160. Tatebayashi Y, Lee MH, Li L, Iqbal K, Grundke-Iqbal I. The dentate gyrus neurogenesis: A therapeutic target for Alzheimer's disease. *Acta Neuropathol (Berl).* 2003;105(3):225–232.

161. Madjid N, Tottie EE, Luttgen M, et al. 5–Hydroxytryptamine 1A receptor blockade facilitates aversive learning in mice: Interactions with cholinergic and glutamatergic mechanisms. *J Pharmacol Exp Ther.* 2006;316(2):581–591. Epub 2005 Oct 13.

162. Bachurin SO, Shevtsova EP, Kireeva EG, et al. Mitochondria as a target for neurotoxins and neuroprotective agents. *Ann N Y Acad Sci.* 2003;993:334–344, discussion 345–349.

163. Doody RS, Gavrilova SI, Sano M, et al. Effect of dimebon on cognition, activities of daily living, behaviour, and global function in patients with mild-to-moderate Alzheimer's disease: A randomized, double blind, placebo-controlled study. *Lancet.* 2008;372(9634):207–215.

164. Wischik CM, Edwards PC, Lai RY, Roth M, Harrington CR. Selective inhibition of Alzheimer disease-like tau aggregation by phenothiazines. *Proc Natl Acad Sci USA.* 1996;93(20):11213–11218.

165. Gura T. Hope in Alzheimer's fight emerges from unexpected places. *Nat Med.* 2008;14(9):894.

166. Namenda [package insert]. St. Louis, MO: Forest Laboratories; 2007.

167. Razadyne / Razadyne ER [package insert]. Titusville, NJ: Ortho-McNeil Neurologics, Inc; 2006.

168. Hill JW, Futterman R, Duttagupta S, et al. Alzheimer's disease and related dementias increase costs of comorbidities in managed Medicare. *Neurology.* 2002;58:62–70.

169. Whitmer RA, Sidney S, Selby J, Johnston SC, Yaffe K. Midlife cardiovascular risk factors and risk of dementia in late life. *Neurology*. 2005;64(2):277–281.

170. Qiu WQ, Folstein MF. Insulin, insulin-degrading enzyme and amyloid-beta peptide in Alzheimer's disease: Review and hypothesis. *Neurobiol Aging*. 2006;27(2):190–198. Epub 2005 Feb 17.

171. Skoog I, Gustafson D. Update on hypertension and Alzheimer's disease. *Neurol Res*. 2006;28(6):605–611.

172. Martins IJ, Hone E, Foster JK, et al. Apolipoprotein E, cholesterol metabolism, diabetes, and the convergence of risk factors for Alzheimer's disease and cardiovascular disease. *Mol Psychiatry*. 2006;11(8):721–736. Epub 2006 Jun 20. Review.

173. Morris MC, Evans DA, Bienias JL, et al. Dietary fats and the risk of incident Alzheimer disease. *Arch Neurol*. 2003;60:194–200.

174. Luchsinger JA, Mayeux R. Dietary factors and Alzheimer's disease. *Lancet Neurol*. 2004;3:579–587.

175. Luchsinger JA, Tang MX, Shea S, Mayeux R. Caloric intake and the risk of Alzheimer's disease. *Arch Neurol*. 2002;59:1258–1263.

176. Hughes TF, Borenstein AR, Schofield E, Wu Y, Larson EB. Association between late-life body mass index and dementia: The Kame Project. *Neurology*. 2009;72(20):1741–1746.

177. Whitmer RA, Gunderson EP, Quesenberry CP Jr, Zhou J, Yaffe K. Body mass index in midlife and risk of Alzheimer disease and vascular dementia. *Curr Alzheimer Res*. 2007;4(2):103–109.

178. Lesser JM, Hughes SV. Psychosis-related disturbances. Psychosis, agitation, and disinhibition in Alzheimer's disease: Definitions and treatment options. *Geriatrics*. 2006;61(12):14–20.

179. Gerber GJ, Prince PN, Snider HG, et al. Group activity and cognitive improvement among patients with Alzheimer's disease. *Hosp Community Psychiatry*. 1991; 42(8):843–845.

180. Karlsson I, Brane G, Melin E, et al. Effects of environmental stimulation on biochemical and physiological variables in dementia. *Acta Psychiatr Scand*. 1998;77(2):207–213.

181. Rovner BW, Steele CD, Shmuely Y, Folstein MF. A randomized trial of dementia care in nursing homes. *J Am Geriatr Soc*. 1996;44(1):7–13.

182. Spector A, Orrell M, Davies S, Woods RT. Can reality orientation be rehabilitated? Developing and piloting of an evidence-based programme of cognition-based therapies for people with dementia. *Neuropsychol Rehabil*. 2001;11:377–379.

183. Teri L, Gallagher-Thompson D. Cognitive-behavioral interventions for treatment of depression in Alzheimer's patients. *Gerontologist*. 1991;31(3):413–416.

184. Teri L, Logsdon RG, Uomoto J, McCurry SM. Behavioral treatment of depression in dementia patients: A controlled clinical trial. *J Gerontol B Psychol Sci Soc Sci*. 1997;52(4):P159–P166.

185. Buettner LL, Fitzsimmons S. AD-venture program: Therapeutic biking for the treatment of depression in long-term care residents with dementia. *Am J Alzheimers Dis Other Demen*. 2002;17(2):121–127.

186. Ashida S. The effect of reminiscence music therapy sessions on changes in depressive symptoms in elderly persons with dementia. *J Music Ther*. 2000;37(3):170–182.

187. Brotons M, Marti P. Music therapy with Alzheimer's patients and their family caregivers: A pilot project. *J Music Ther.* 2003;40(2): 138–150.

188. Kydd P. Using music therapy to help a client with Alzheimer's disease adapt to long-term care. *Am J Alzheimers Dis Other Demen.* 2001;16(2):103–108.

189. Kipling T, Bailey M, Charlesworth G. The feasibility of a cognitive behavioral therapy group for men with mild/moderate cognitive impairment. *Behav Cognit Psychother.* 1999;27:189–193.

190. Haupt M, Karger A, Janner M. Improvement of agitation and anxiety in demented patients after psychoeducative group intervention with their caregivers. *Int J Geriatr Psychiatry.* 2000;15(12):1125–1129.

191. Brane G, Karlsson I, Kihlgren M, Nordberg A. Integrity-promoting care of demented nursing home patients: Psychological and biochemical changes. *Int J Geriatr Psychiatry.* 1989;4:165–172.

192. Svansdottir HB, Snaedal J. Music therapy in moderate and severe dementia of Alzheimer's type: A case-control study. *Int Psychogeriatr.* 2006;18(4):613–621. Epub 2006 Apr 18.

193. Coltharp W Jr, Richie MF, Kaas MJ. Wandering. *J Gerontol Nurs.* 1996;22(11):5–10.

194. Heard K, Watson TS. Reducing wandering by persons with dementia using differential reinforcement. *J Appl Behav Anal.* 1999;32(3):381–384.

195. Dickinson JI, McLain-Kark J, Marshall-Baker A. The effects of visual barriers on exiting behavior in a dementia care unit. *Gerontologist.* 1995;35(1):127–130.

196. Namazi KH, Johnson BD. Pertinent autonomy for residents with dementias: modification of the physical environment to enhance independence. *Am J Alzheimer's Care and Related Disorders and Research.* 1992;7:16–21.

197. Hewawasam L. Floor patterns limit wandering of people with Alzheimer's. *Nurs Times.* 1996;92(22):41–44.

198. Politis AM, Vozzella S, Mayer LS, et al. A randomized, controlled, clinical trial of activity therapy for apathy in patients with dementia residing in long-term care. *Int J Geriatr Psychiatry.* 2004;19(11):1087–1094.

199. Lesser JM, Hughes SV. Psychosis-related disturbances. Psychosis, agitation, and disinhibition in Alzheimer's disease: Definitions and treatment options. *Geriatrics* 2006 Nov; 61 (11): 14–20.

200. Rogers JC, Holm MB, Burgio LD, et al. Improving morning care routines of nursing home residents with dementia. *J Am Geriatr Soc.* 1999;47(9):1049–1057.

201. Bakke BL, Kvale S, Burns T, et al. Multicomponent intervention for agitated behavior in a person with Alzheimer's disease. *J Appl Behav Anal.* 1994;27(1):175–176.

202. Moniz-Cook E, Woods RT, Richards K. Functional analysis of challenging behaviour in dementia: The role of superstition. *Int J Geriatr Psychiatry.* 2001;16(1):45–56.

203. Snyder M, Egan EC, Burns KR. Efficacy of hand massage in decreasing agitation behaviors associated with care activities in persons with dementia. *Geriatr Nurs.* 1995;16(2):60–63.

204. Gerdner LA. Use of individualized music by trained staff and family: Translating research into practice. *J Gerontol Nurs.* 2005;31(6):22–30, quiz 55–56.

205. Baker R, Bell S, Baker E, et al. A randomized controlled trial of the effects of multi-sensory stimulation (MSS) for people with dementia. *Br J Clin Psychol.* 2001;40(part 1):81–96.

206. Baker R, Dowling Z, Wareing LA, et al. Snoezelen: Its long-term and short-term effects on older people with dementia. *Br J Occupational Therapy.* 1997;60:213–218.

207. Camberg L, Woods P, Ooi WL, et al. Evaluation of simulated presence: A personalized approach to enhance well-being in persons with Alzheimer's disease. *J Am Geriatr Soc.* 1999;47(4):446–452.

208. Cohen-Mansfield J. Non-pharmacological interventions for psychotic symptoms in dementia. *J Geriatr Psychiatry Neurol.* 2003;16:219–224.

209. Kidder SW. Psychosis in the elderly—whose delusion is it? *Geriatr Times.* 2003;4(2):25–26.

210. Hall L, Hare J. Video respite for cognitively impaired persons in nursing homes. *Am J Alzheimer Dis Other Dement.* 1997;12(3): 117–121.

211. Satlin A, Volicer L, Ross V, et al. Bright light treatment of behavioral and sleep disturbances in patients with Alzheimer's disease. *Am J Psychiatry.* 1992;149(8):1028–1032.

212. Lindenmuth GF, Patel M, Chang PK. Effects of music on sleep in healthy elderly and subjects with senile dementia of the Alzheimer's type. *Am J Alzheimer Care Related Disord Res.* 1992;7:13–20.

213. McCurry SM, Logsdon RG, Vitiello MV, Teri L. Treatment of sleep and nighttime disturbances in Alzheimer's disease: A behavior management approach. *Sleep Med.* 2004;5(4):373–377.

214. McCurry SM, Gibbons LE, Logsdon RG, et al. Nighttime insomnia treatment and education for Alzheimer's disease: A randomized, controlled trial. *J Am Geriatr Soc.* 2005;53(5):793–802.

215. Woods B, Spector A, Jones C, et al. Reminiscence therapy for dementia. *Cochrane Database Syst Rev.* 2005;2:CD001120. Review.

216. Neal M, Briggs M. Validation therapy for dementia. *Cochrane Database Syst Rev.* 2003;3:CD001394.

217. Spector A, Orrell M, Davies S, Woods B. Reality orientation for dementia. *Cochrane Database Syst Rev.* 2000;4:CD001119.

218. Gillick MR. Rethinking the role of tube feeding in patients with advanced dementia. *N Engl J Med.* 2000;342(3):206–210.

219. Finucane TE, Bynum JP. Use of tube feeding to prevent aspiration pneumonia. *Lancet.* 1996;348:1421–1424.

220. Finucane TE, Christmas C, Travis K. Tube feeding in patients with advanced dementia: A review of the evidence. *JAMA.* 1999;282(14):1365–1370.

221. Kaw M, Sekas G. Long-term follow-up of consequences of percutaneous endoscopic gastrostomy (PEG) tubes in nursing home patients. *Dig Dis Sci.* 1994;39:738–743.

222. Aupperle PM, MacPhee ER, Strozeski JE, et al. Hospice use for the patient with advanced Alzheimer's disease: The role of the geriatric psychiatrist. *Am J Hosp Palliative Care.* 2004;21:427–437.

223. Overman W Jr, Stoudemire A. Guidelines for legal and financial counseling of Alzheimer's disease patients and their families. *Am J Psychiatry.* 1988;145(12):1495–1500.

224. Zimny GH, Grossberg GT, eds. *Guardianship of the Aged: Medical, Legal and Judicial Aspects.* New York: Springer Publishing Co; 1998.

225. Marson DC, Schmitt FA, Ingram KK, et al. Determining the competency of Alzheimer patients to consent to treatment and research. *Alzheimer Dis Assoc Disord.* 1994;8(suppl 4):5–18.

226. Chard LP, Kirkendall JN. Guardianships and conservatorships. In: *Advising the Older Client.* Ann Arbor MI: Institute of Continuing Legal Education; 1990 (revised 1993):717–792.

227. Ory MG, Hoffman RR 3rd, Yee JL, Tennstedt S, Schulz R. Prevalence and impact of caregiving: A detailed comparison between dementia and nondementia caregivers. *Gerontologist.* 1999;39(2):177–185.

228. Schulz R, O'Brien AT, Bookwala J, Fleissner K. Psychiatric and physical morbidity effects of dementia caregiving: Prevalence, correlates, and causes. *Gerontologist.* 1995;35:771–791.

229. Robinson-Whelen S, Tada Y, MacCallum RC, McGuire L, Kiecolt-Glaser JK. Long-term caregiving: What happens when it ends? *J Abnorm Psychol.* 2001;110:573–584

230. Mittelman MS, Haley WE, Clay OJ, Roth DL. Improving caregiver well-being delays nursing home placement of patients with Alzheimer disease. *Neurology.* 2006;67(9):1592–1599.

231. Mittelman MS, Roth DL, Coon DW, et al. Sustained benefit of supportive intervention for depressive symptoms in caregivers of patients with Alzheimer's disease. *Am J Psychiatry.* 2004;161:850–856.

232. Smith GE, Kokmen E, O'Brien PC. Risk factors for nursing home placement in a population-based dementia cohort. *J Am Geriatr Soc.* 2000;48(5):519–525.

233. Buhr GT, Kuchibhatla M, Clipp EC. Caregivers' reasons for nursing home placement: Clues for improving discussions with families prior to the transition. *Gerontologist.* 2006;46(1):52–61.

234. Balestreri L, Grossberg A, Grossberg GT. Behavioral and psychological symptoms of dementia as a risk factor for nursing home placement. *Int Psychogeriatr.* 2000;12(suppl 1):59–62.

235. Holmes D, Teresi J, Weiner A, et al. Impact associated with special care units in long-term care facilities. *Gerontologist.* 1990;30:178–181.

Index

A

Acetylcholine, 34
Acetylcholinesterase, 36
Activities of daily living, 10
    adult daycare services and, 81
    Alzheimer's disease and loss in capacity for, 1
    Barthel ADL Index and, 20–21
    differentiating stages of Alzheimer's disease and, 5*t*
    difficulties with, 11, 13, 15*t*
    integrity-promoting care and, 64
    responses to antidementia therapy and, 41*t*
    severe Alzheimer's disease and, 4
AD. *See* Alzheimer's disease
ADAS. *See* Alzheimer's Disease Assessment Scale
ADLs. *See* Activities of daily living
ADRD. *See* Alzheimer's disease and related dementias
Adult daycare services, 80–81, 83*t*
Advance directives, 75–76, 84
Age
    Alzheimer's disease risk and, 6
    memory impairment associated with, 29
Aggression, 1, 4, 14, 15*t*
Agitation, 13, 14, 15*t*, 66–67
Agnosia, 2, 4, 12, 13, 15*t*
Alcohol, moderate intake, protection against AD and, 8, 10
Allele, 6
Allosteric modulation, 36
Alzheimer's Association, 39
Alzheimer's disease
    affect of, on patient's lives, 3–4
    assessing, 11
    brain areas involved in, 34–35
    clinical assessment of, 18–27
    comorbidity and pharmacotherapy choices for, 56–58
    defined, 2–3
    diagnosis of, 32
    diagnostic criteria for, 14, 16, 17, 18
    diagnostic workup summary for, 28*t*
    differentiating normal aging from, 27–31
    differentiating stages of, by domain, 5*t*
    DSM-IV-TR criteria for, 16*t*, 32
    economic toll related to, 2, 10, 57
    emerging or disease-modifying treatments for, 52–56
    incidence of, 5
    lifestyle modifications and preventive measures in, 58–59
    medications for
        behavioral and psychological symptoms of dementia, 45–50
        stabilization or improvement of symptoms, 35–45
        summary of, with dosages and side effects, 40*t*
    neuroanatomical and neurochemical hallmarks of, 34–35
    NINCDS-ADRDA criteria for, 16*t*, 32
    Parkinson disease dementia *vs.*, 30
    presenting features with, 11–14
        activities of daily living, 13
        behavior, 13–14
        cognition, 12–13
    protective factors against, 8–10, 10*t*
    psychosocial interventions for patients with, 61–69
        agitation, 66–67
        anxiety, 63–64
        apathy, 65–66
        depression, 62–63
        psychosis, 67–69
        sleep abnormalities, 69
        wandering, 64–65
    responses to antidementia therapy by domain at stages of, 41*t*
    risk factors for, 6–8, 10, 10*t*
    stages in, 1, 3–4, 5*t*
    summary of deficits in, 15*t*
    treatment recommendations for, 39
    vaccine against, 54–55
Alzheimer's disease and related dementias
    comorbidities in, 58
    economic toll related to, 57
Alzheimer's Disease Assessment Scale, 26
Amygdala, 34, 35
Amyloid, 2
Amyloid angiopathy, 3
Amyloid imaging, 23
Amyloid-modifying agents, 53–54
Amyloid plaques, 23
Amyloid precursor protein, 6
Antibiotics, end-of-life care and, 73–74
Anticonvulsants, 48–49
Antidepressant medications, 48
Anti-inflammatory drugs, 8, 53. *See also* Tarenflurbil
Antipsychotics, 45–47
    atypical/second generation, 45–47
    typical/conventional, 47
Anxiety, 14, 63–64
Apathy, 65–66
Aphasia, 2, 12, 15*t*
APOE2, 6, 7, 8
APOE4, 10, 23, 59